Blueprints
SURGERY

FOURTH EDITION

Blueprints
SURGERY

FOURTH EDITION

Seth J. Karp, MD
Attending Surgeon
Beth Israel Deaconess Medical Center
Assistant Professor of Surgery
Harvard Medical School
Boston, Massachusetts

James P. G. Morris, MD
Thoracic and General Surgeon
The Permanente Medical Group
South San Francisco Kaiser Hospital
South San Francisco, California

Questions and answers provided by

Stanley Zaslau, MD, MBA, FACS
Associate Professor
Division of Urology
West Virginia University
School of Medicine
Morgantown, West Virginia

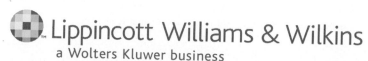

Lippincott Williams & Wilkins
a Wolters Kluwer business

Philadelphia • Baltimore • New York • London
Buenos Aires • Hong Kong • Sydney • Tokyo

Acquisitions Editor: Nancy Anastasi Duffy
Managing Editor: Kathleen H. Scogna
Marketing Manager: Jennifer Kuklinski
Associate Production Manager: Kevin P. Johnson
Creative Director: Doug Smock
Compositor: International Typesetting and Composition
Printer: Quebecor World Dubuque

Library of Congress Cataloging-in-Publication Data

Karp, Seth J.
  Blueprints surgery / Seth J. Karp, James P.G. Morris; questions and answers provided by Stanley Zaslau.—4th ed.
       p. ; cm.—(Blueprints)
  Includes bibliographical references and index.
  ISBN 1-4051-0499-6
  1. Surgery—Outlines, syllabi, etc.   I. Morris, James, 1964-   II. Zaslau, Stanley.   III. Title.   IV. Series.
  [DNLM: 1. Surgical Procedures, Operative—Examination Questions. WO 18.2 K18b 2006]
  RD37.3.K37 2006
  617'.910076—dc22   2006004933

Dedication

To Lauren, Sarah, and Jay. S.J.K.

To Caroline, Isabel, Grant, and Cameron. J.P.G.M.

Preface

In 1997, the first five books in the *Blueprints* series were published as board review for medical students, interns, and residents who wanted high-yield, accurate clinical content for U.S. Medical Licensing Examination Steps 2 and 3. Nine years later, we are proud to report that the original books and the entire *Blueprints* brand of review materials have far exceeded our expectations.

Significant expansion of the material distinguishes the fourth addition. Four new chapters have been added: an introductory chapter on techniques, a chapter on plastic surgery, a chapter on orthopedic surgery, and a chapter on perioperative care. Sample operative reports are included in an appendix. Similar to previous editions, the entire text has been updated. As *Blueprints* is used in a wider range of clinical settings, students commented that additional material would be useful. In response, an increased number of figures, including radiographic studies, photographs, and drawings, integrate with the text. Suggestions for additional reading appear at the end of each chapter for students wanting more detail on a particular subject. These references have been carefully chosen to provide state-of-the-art information, and much of this material has been published within the past two years. Finally, completely new questions reflect the current format of the Boards.

We sincerely hope this edition preserves the original vision of *Blueprints* to provide concise, useful information for students and that the additional material enhances this vision.

Contents

Abbreviations

ABGs	arterial blood gases
ACAS	Asymptomatic Carotid Atherosclerosis Study
ACE	angiotensin-converting enzyme
ACTH	adrenocorticotropic hormone
ADH	antidiuretic hormone
AFP	alpha-fetoprotein
AI	aortic insufficiency
ALT	alanine transaminase
ANA	antinuclear antibody
AP	anteroposterior
APKD	adult polycystic kidney disease
ARDS	adult respiratory distress syndrome
AS	aortic stenosis
ASD	atrial septal defect
AST	aspartate transaminase
ATLS	Advanced Trauma Life Support
AUA-IPSS	American Urological Association Symptom Score
AV	arteriovenous
BCC	basal cell carcinoma
BCG	bacill (bacillus) Calmette-Guérin
BE	barium enema
β-hCG	beta-human chorionic gonadotropin
BP	blood pressure
BPH	benign prostatic hypertrophy
BRCA	breast cancer gene
BUN	blood urea nitrogen
CABG	coronary artery bypass graft
CAD	coronary artery disease
CBC	complete blood count
CCK	cholecystokinin
CDC	Centers for Disease Control and Prevention
CEA	carcinoembryonic antigen
CES	cauda equina syndrome
CHF	congestive heart failure
CIS	carcinoma in situ
CMF	cyclophosphamide, methotrexate, and 5-fluorouracil
CMV	cytomegalovirus
CN	cranial nerve
CNS	central nervous system
COPD	chronic obstructive pulmonary disease
CPAP	continuous positive airway pressure
CRF	corticotropin-releasing factor
CRH	corticotropin-releasing hormone
CSF	cerebrospinal fluid
CT	computed tomography
CXR	chest x-ray
DCIS	ductal carcinoma in situ
DEXA	dual-energy x-ray absorptiometry
DHT	dihydrotestosterone
DIC	disseminated intravascular coagulation
DIP	distal interphalangeal
DNA	deoxyribonucleic acid
DTRs	deep tendon reflexes
EEG	electroencephalogram
EGD	esophagogastroduodenoscopy
EKG	electrocardiography
EMG	electromyography
ERCP	endoscopic retrograde cholangiopancreatography
ESR	erythrocyte sedimentation rate
EUS	endoscopic esophageal ultrasound
ESWL	extracorporeal shock wave lithotripsy
FDG-PET	fluorodeoxyglucose positron emission tomography
FNA	fine-needle aspiration
FSH	follicle-stimulating hormone
G-6-PD	glucose-6-phosphate dehydrogenase
GBM	glioblastoma multiforme
GCS	Glasgow Coma Scale
GERD	gastroesophageal reflux disease
GGT	gamma-glutamyl transferase
GH	growth hormone
GI	gastrointestinal
GU	genitourinary
Hb	hemoglobin
hCG	human chorionic gonadotropin
HIDA	hepatobiliary iminodiacetic acid
HIV	human immunodeficiency virus
HLA	human leukocyte antigen
HPF	high-power field
HPI	history of present illness
HPV	human papilloma virus
HR	heart rate
ICP	intracranial pressure
ID/CC	identification and chief complaint

IgA	immunoglobulin A
IL-2	interleukin-2
IMA	inferior mesenteric artery
IMV	inferior mesenteric vein
INR	international normalized ratio
ITP	immune thrombocytopenic purpura
IVP	intravenous pyelography
JVD	jugular venous distention
KUB	kidneys/ureter/bladder
LAD	left anterior descending coronary artery
LCA	left coronary artery
LCIS	lobular carcinoma in situ
LCX	left circumflex
LDH	lactate dehydrogenase
LES	lower esophageal sphincter
LFTs	liver function tests
LH	luteinizing hormone
LH-RH	luteinizing hormone-releasing hormone
LM	left main coronary artery
LVH	left ventricular hypertrophy
Lytes	electrolytes
MCP	metacarpophalangeal
MCV	mean corpuscular volume
MELD	Model for End-Stage Liver Disease
MEN	multiple endocrine neoplasia
MHC	major histocompatibility complex
MI	myocardial infarction
MMF	mycophenolate mofetil
MPA	mycophenolic acid
MR	mitral regurgitation
MRCP	magnetic resonance cholangiopancreatography
MRI	magnetic resonance imaging
MS	mitral stenosis
MTC	medullary thyroid carcinoma
MVA	motor vehicle accident
NASCET	North American Symptomatic Carotid Endarterectomy Trial
NG	nasogastric
NPO	nil per os (nothing by mouth)
NSAID	nonsteroidal anti-inflammatory drug
NSGCT	nonseminomatous germ cell tumor
Nuc	nuclear medicine
OPSS	overwhelming postsplenectomy sepsis
PA	posteroanterior
PBS	peripheral blood smear
PCNL	percutaneous nephrolithotomy
PDA	posterior descending coronary artery
PDS	polydioxanone
PE	physical examination
PEEP	positive end-expiratory pressure
PET	positron-emission tomography
PFTs	pulmonary function tests

PIP	proximal interphalangeal
PMI	point of maximal impulse
PP	pancreatic polypeptide
PPI	proton-pump inhibitors
PSA	prostate-specific antigen
PT	prothrombin time
PTC	percutaneous transhepatic cholangiography
PTH	parathyroid hormone
PTU	propylthiouracil
RA	right atrium
RBC	red blood cell
RCA	right coronary artery
REM	rapid eye movement
RPLND	retroperitoneal lymph node dissection
RR	respiratory rate
RV	right ventricular
RVH	right ventricular hypertrophy
SAH	subarachnoid hemorrhage
SBFT	small bowel follow-through
SBO	small bowel obstruction
SCC	squamous cell carcinoma
SIADH	syndrome of inappropriate secretion of ADH
SLNB	sentinel lymph node biopsy
SMA	superior mesenteric artery
SMV	superior mesenteric vein
SSI	surgical site infection
STD	sexually transmitted disease
STSG	split-thickness skin graft
TCC	transitional cell carcinoma
TIA	transient ischemic attack
TIBC	total iron-binding capacity
TIPS	transjugular intrahepatic portosystemic shunt
TNM	tumors, nodes, metastases classification
TPN	total parenteral nutrition
TRAM	transverse rectus abdominis myocutaneous
TRH	thyrotropin-releasing hormone
TSH	thyroid-stimulating hormone
TUBD	transurethral balloon dilatation
TUNA	transurethral needle ablation
TURP	transurethral resection of the prostate
UA	urinalysis
UGI	upper gastrointestinal
US	ultrasound
UTI	urinary tract infection
UV	ultraviolet
VMA	vanillylmandelic acid
VS	vital signs
VSD	ventricular septal defect
WBC	white blood cell
XR	x-ray

Surgical Techniques

INTRODUCTION

As with most endeavors in life, the healing arts are divided into both the theoretical and the practical spheres. Surgeons are fortunate to practice equally in both spheres by applying their intellect and technical skill to the diagnosis and treatment of sickness. The practice of surgery is unique in the realm of medicine and correspondingly carries added responsibilities. Patients literally place their trust in the hands of surgeons. The profound nature of cutting into another human being, and artfully manipulating his or her physical being to achieve wellness, requires reverence, skill, and judgment.

Technologic advances in modern medicine have led to the rise and establishment of procedure-related specialties, including invasive cardiology and radiology, dermatology, intensive care medicine and emergency medicine, to name a few. Manipulative skills are now required not only in the operating room but also in procedure rooms and emergency rooms for invasive treatments and repairing traumatic injuries. Therefore medical students and residents should master the basics of surgical technique so they are well prepared for the challenges ahead.

PREOPERATIVE ISSUES

For well-trained and experienced surgeons, performing an operation is usually a routine affair and is relatively simple. One of the difficulties in taking care of surgical patients, however, is actually making the decision to operate. Operating is simple; deciding not to operate is the more difficult decision. Once the decision has been made to proceed with surgery, always have a clear operative plan and prepare for any potential deviations that may be required based on the intraoperative findings.

A thorough discussion with the patient is required before deciding to operate, to outline the clinical situation and indications for surgery. All reasonable management options should be reviewed and the risks and potential complications of each presented. Appropriate written approval must be obtained—usually a "request" for operation, rather than a more passive "consent"—and signed by the patient or guardian, the person performing the procedure, and a witness.

Adequate preparation of a patient for surgery depends on the intended operation and the patient's general condition. Elderly patients with multiple medical problems should be evaluated thoroughly and their health status maximized. Preoperative consultations with a cardiologist, diabetologist, or internist may be necessary.

To prevent surgical site infections (SSI), various techniques are employed. Prior to colon surgery, mechanical and chemical cleansing of the large intestine is typical to decrease bacterial counts. Preoperative showers can be used to decrease the bacterial count of the skin. Regarding hair removal, no hair removal is preferred: The Centers for Disease Control and Prevention (CDC) guidelines for hair removal state that only the interfering hair around the incision site should be removed, if necessary. Removal should be done immediately before the operation, preferably with electric clippers. Using electric clippers minimizes microscopic skin cuts, which are more common from traditional blade razors and which serve as foci for bacterial multiplication. Giving preoperative intravenous antibiotics shortly before the initial incision and maintaining patient core temperature to avoid hypothermia are standard practices. CDC guidelines also advise diagnosis and treatment of "all infections remote to the surgical site before elective

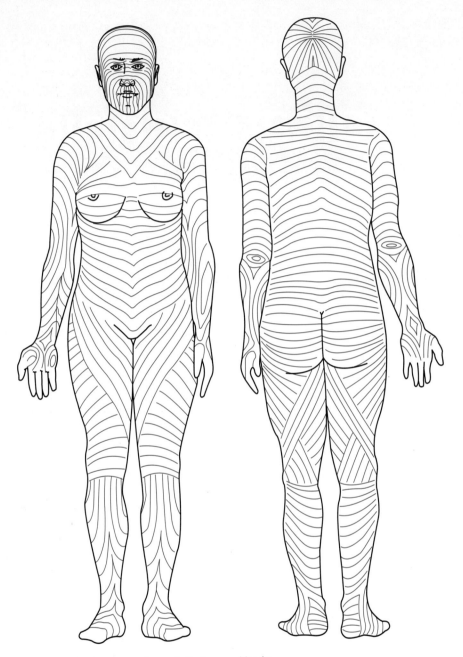

Figure 1-1 • Skin tension lines of the face and body.
Adapted from Simon R, Brenner B. *Procedures and Techniques in Emergency Medicine*. Baltimore, MD: Williams & Wilkins; 1982.

■ **TABLE 1-1** Pharmacologic Properties of Local Anesthetic Agents					
Agent	**Concentration**	**Onset of Action**		**Duration of Action**	**Maximum Allowable Dose One Time**
		Infiltration	**Block**		
Lidocaine (Xylocaine)	1.0%	Immediate	4–10 min	60–120 min (for blocks)	4.5 mg/kg of 1% (30 cc per average adult)
Bupivacaine (Marcaine)	0.25%	Slower	8–12 min	240–480 min (for blocks)	3 mg/kg of 0.25% (50 cc per average adult)

Adapted from Trott A. Wounds and Lacerations: Emergency Care and Closure. *2nd ed. St. Louis, MO: Mosby–Year Book; 1997:31.*

operation and postpone elective operations on patients with remote site infections until the infection has resolved."

To minimize surgical misadventure, most hospitals have borrowed techniques from the aviation industry, instituting routines that call for preoperative surgical site marking and verification.

INTRAOPERATIVE ISSUES

Before beginning the operation, ensure the overall operating room environment is to your satisfaction. The operating table and overhead lights should be correctly positioned. Room temperature and ambient noise should be adjusted as necessary. Play music if appropriate. Ensure adequate positioning and prepping of the patient and communicate with the anesthesiologist and operating room team to confirm readiness. Then scrub, gown, and drape. Prior to incision—again to minimize surgical misadventure—many hospitals call for a final check to ensure that the correct patient is undergoing the correct procedure.

Deciding where to make the skin incision is usually straightforward; however, knowledge of the skin's intrinsic tension lines is important to maximize wound healing and cosmesis. Incisions made parallel to the natural lines of tension usually heal with thinner scars because the static and dynamic forces on the wound are minimized. When making elective facial skin excisions or repairs of traumatic facial lacerations, keep in mind that incisions perpendicular to these tension lines will result in wider, less cosmetically acceptable scars (Fig. 1-1).

Although general anesthetic techniques are usually the anesthesiologist's job, all invasive practitioners should have a working knowledge of local anesthetics. Depending on the procedure being performed, the choice of local anesthetic must be tailored to each patient. Local anesthetics diffuse across nerve membranes and interfere with neural depolarization and transmission. Each local anesthetic agent has a different onset of action, duration of activity, and toxicity. Epinephrine is often administered concurrently with the local anesthetic agent to induce vasoconstriction, thereby prolonging the duration of action and decreasing bleeding. The two most commonly used local anesthetics are the shorter-acting lidocaine (Xylocaine) and the longer-acting bupivacaine (Marcaine), the properties of which are outlined in Table 1-1.

Lidocaine (1% and 2%, with and without epinephrine) has a rapid onset of action, achieving sensory block in 4 to 10 minutes. The duration of action is about 75 minutes (60 to 120 minutes). The maximum allowable dosage is 4.5 mg/kg/dose without epinephrine or 7 mg/kg/dose with epinephrine.

Bupivacaine (0.25%, 0.5%, and 0.75%, with and without epinephrine) has a slower onset of action, taking 8 to 12 minutes for a simple block. Duration of action is approximately four times longer than lidocaine, lasting 2 to 8 hours, making bupivacaine the preferred agent for longer procedures and for prolonged action. The maximum allowable dosage is 3 mg/kg/dose.

INSTRUMENTS

The basic tools of a surgeon are a knife for cutting and a needle with suture for restoring tissues to their appropriate position and function. Additional tools and instrumentation simply allow operations to be performed with greater finesse.

The most commonly used knife blades are illustrated in Figure 1-2 and are made functional by attachment to a standard no. 3 Bard-Parker knife handle. Choose the size and shape of the blade based on the intended indication. Abdominal or thoracic skin incisions are typically made with no. 10, 20, or 22 blades, whereas more delicate incisions could require the smaller no. 15 blade. The sharp-tipped no. 11 blade is ideal for entering and draining an abscess or for making an

BARD-PARKER

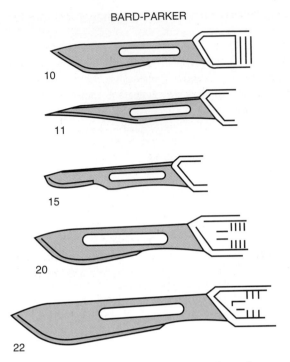

10

11

15

20

22

Figure 1-2 • General surgery knife blades. Shown here are Bard-Parker no. 10, 11, 15, 20, and 22 with attached handles.
Adapted from Malt R. *The Practice of Surgery.* Philadelphia, PA: WB Saunders; 1993:17.

arteriotomy by incising a blood vessel in preparation for vascular procedures.

Scissors are mainly used for dissecting and cutting tissues. All scissors are designed for right-handed use. Each pair of scissors should only be used for the indication for which it was designed (Fig. 1-3). Most scissors have either straight or curved tips. Fine iris scissors are used for delicate dissection and cutting. Metzenbaum scissors are versatile, general-use instruments. Sturdy Mayo scissors are used for cutting thick or dense tissues, such as fascia, scar, or tendons.

Various forceps have been developed to facilitate manipulation of objects within the operative field, as well as to stabilize tissues and assist in dissection. All forceps perform essentially the same function but differ in the design of their tips and their intrinsic delicacy of form (Fig. 1-4). Toothed forceps are useful for stabilizing and moving tissues, whereas smooth atraumatic forceps are more appropriate for delicate vascular manipulation. DeBakey forceps are good general-use instruments with atraumatic flat tips and tiny fine serrations. Fine-toothed Adson forceps are ideal for skin closure, and stout-toothed Bonney forceps are excellent for facial closure.

Needle and suture are used to maintain tissue apposition until healing has occurred. The array of needles and suture material is vast; therefore, the surgeon's choice is based on the specific indication at hand.

Needles come either straight or curved. Curved needles are usually half circle or three-eighths circle. Sewing in a deep hole may require a five-eighths circle

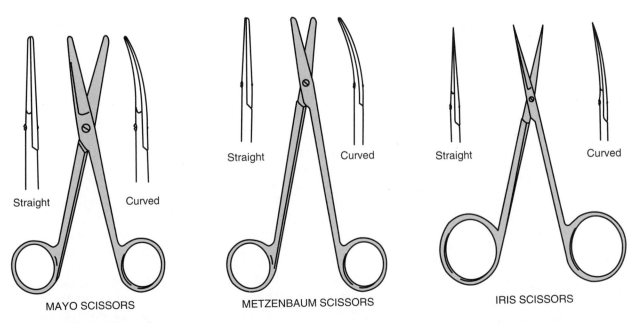

Straight Curved

Straight Curved

Straight Curved

MAYO SCISSORS

METZENBAUM SCISSORS

IRIS SCISSORS

Figure 1-3 • Mayo, Metzenbaum, and iris scissors.
Adapted from Van Way C, Buerk C. *Pocket Manual of Basic Surgical Skills.* St. Louis: CV Mosby; 1986:14–15.

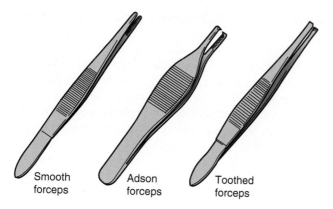

Figure 1-4 • Smooth, Adson, and toothed forceps.
Adapted from Van Way C, Buerk C. *Pocket Manual of Basic Surgical Skills.* St. Louis, MO: CV Mosby; 1986:18.

needle, whereas microsurgery often requires quarter circle needles.

The needle can have an eye for threading the suture (French eye), or the needle has an already attached suture (swaged). Most needles today are swaged, meaning they are a needle-suture combination. Etymologically, a swage is a blacksmithing tool used to shape metal. Thus, a swaged needle is manufactured by placing the suture into the hollow shank of a needle and then compressing the needle around the suture, holding it firm. Some sutures are swaged to needles in such a manner that they pop off if excess tension is applied between suture and needle.

Needle tips are either tapered or cutting. Tapered needles are circumferentially smooth and slide between the elements of tissues, whereas cutting needles are triangular in cross section and cut through tissues like a tiny knife (Fig. 1-5).

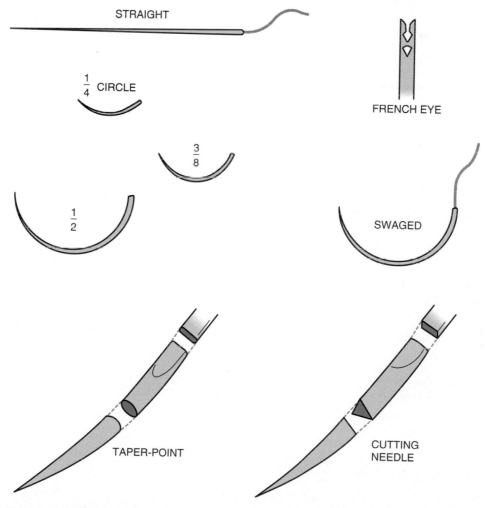

Figure 1-5 • Needle characteristics.
Adapted from Malt R. *The Practice of Surgery.* Philadelphia, PA: WB Saunders; 1993:19.

Suture material is categorized as to its permanence (absorbable or nonabsorbable), its structure (braided or monofilament), and its caliber (Table 1-2).

Absorbable suture material is made from either naturally derived, collagen-based materials or synthetic polymers. Examples of absorbable suture material are gut (plain and chromic), polyglactic acid (Vicryl), polyglycolic acid (Dexon), polyglyconate (Maxon), and polydioxanone (PDS). The suture is either hydrolyzed by water or undergoes enzymatic digestion, thereby losing tensile strength over time.

Permanent nonabsorbable sutures are made from materials impervious to significant chemical degradation and are useful for maintaining long-term tissue apposition. Examples of permanent nonabsorbable suture material are nylon, polypropylene, stainless steel, and silk.

■ TABLE 1-2 Common Suture Material

Material		Loss of Tensile Strength	Inflammatory Reaction	Absorbed	Common Uses
Absorbable					
Gut					Superficial vessels; closure of tissues that heal rapidly (buccal mucosa) and require minimal support
Plain	Sheep intestine	7–10 d	Moderate	2 mo	
Chromic	Treated with chromium salt	10–14 d	Moderate but less	3 mo	
Polyglactic acid (Vicryl); polyglycolic acid (Dexon)	Synthetic polyfilament	4–5 wk	Minimal	3 mo	Dermis; fat muscle
Polyglyconate (Maxon, Monocryl)	Synthetic monofilament	3–4 wk	Minimal	3–4 mo	Subcuticular close and soft tissue approximation
Polydioxanone (PDS)	Synthetic monofilament	8 wk	Minimal	6 mo	Muscle; fascia
Nonabsorbable					
Polypropylene (Prolene)	Polymer of propylene	Years*	Minimal	—	Fascia; muscle; vessels
Nylon (Surgilon, Nurolon)	Polyamide	Years*	Minimal	—	Skin; drains; microsurgical anastomoses
Silk	Raw silk spun by silk worm	1 y	Intense	—	Tie off vessels; bowel
Staples	Iron- chromium- nickel	—	Minimal	—	Skin

*With reoperation, polypropylene and nylon remain present but decompose slightly.
From Taylor JA. Blueprints Plastic Surgery. Malden, MA: Blackwell Science; 2005.

CLOSURE TECHNIQUES

There are many techniques for closing wounds (Fig. 1-6). Wounds can be closed using a continuous stitch that is quick to perform and that results in tension distributed along the length of the suture. Simple interrupted stitching allows for precise tissue approximation (skin or fascia). Mattress stitches can be placed either vertically or horizontally, allowing excellent skin apposition and eversion while minimizing tension. Subcuticular stitching using an absorbable suture at the dermal-epidermal junction is a convenient skin-closure technique, allowing epidermal apposition so that postoperative suture removal is unnecessary. Regardless of the closure technique used, certain basic principles must be considered to avoid wound breakdown and to achieve a well-healed cosmetically satisfactory scar:

• skin incision along intrinsic tension lines
• gentle handling of intraoperative tissue
• meticulous hemostasis
• tension-free closure
• eversion of skin edges

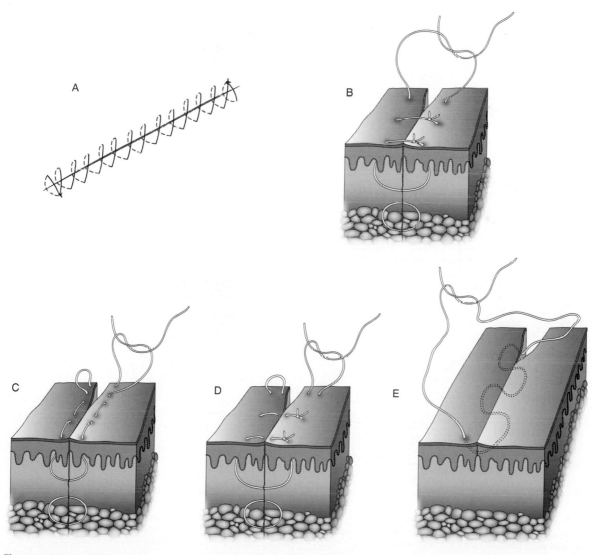

Figure 1-6 • Suturing techniques: **(A)** Continuous, **(B)** simple interrupted, **(C)** horizontal mattress, **(D)** vertical mattress, and **(E)** subcuticular.
From Taylor JA. *Blueprints Plastic Surgery.* Malden, MA: Blackwell Publishing; 2005:7.

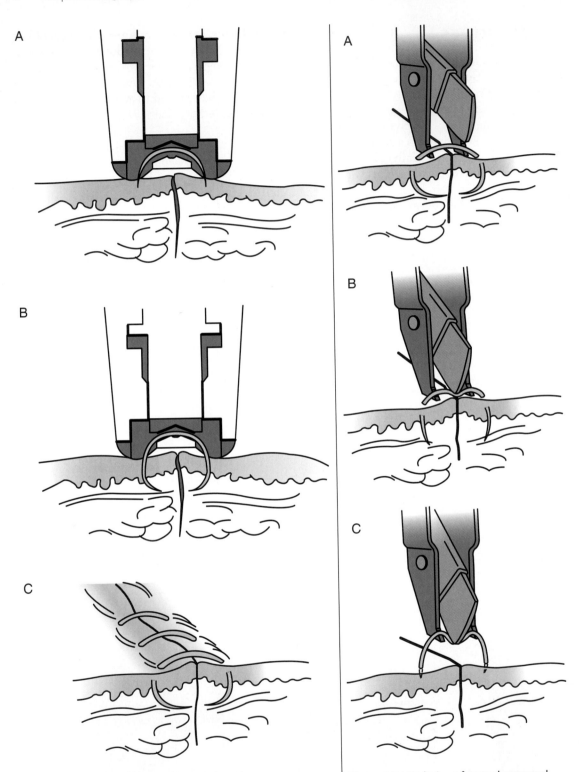

Figure 1-7 • Wound closure using metal staples.
Adapted from Alexander Trott, MD. *Wounds and Lacerations: Emergency Care and Closure.* 2nd ed. St. Louis, MO: Mosby–Year Book; 1997:224.

Figure 1-8 • Technique for staple removal.
From Alexander Trott, MD. *Wounds and Lacerations: Emergency Care and Closure.* 2nd ed. St. Louis, MO: Mosby–Year Book; 1997:225.

An alternative to sutured skin closure of wounds is skin apposition using metal staples. Many elective surgical wounds are closed with skin staples, because the technique allows for rapid skin closure, minimal wound inflammatory response, and near-equivalent cosmetic results. This technique usually works best with two operators: one to evert and align the skin edges with forceps and another to fire the stapler (Fig. 1-7).

Removal of staples is performed using a simple handheld device that deforms the staple and reconfigures the staple shape, allowing for smooth, easy withdrawal (Fig. 1-8).

References

Crabtree TD. *BRS General Surgery*. Philadelphia, PA: Lippincott Williams & Wilkins; 2000.

Wind GG, Rich NM. *Principles of Surgical Technique: The Art of Surgery*. Philadelphia, PA: JB Lippincott; 1987.

Vascular Surgery

ANEURYSMS AND DISSECTIONS

An aneurysm is an abnormal dilation of an artery. Saccular aneurysms occur when a portion of the artery forms an outpouching, or "mushroom." Fusiform aneurysms occur when the entire arterial diameter grows. True aneurysms involve all layers of the arterial wall: intima, media, and adventitia. An artery is considered aneurysmal if the diameter is greater than 1.5 times its normal size. Otherwise an enlarged artery is considered ectatic.

In contrast, a dissection occurs when a defect in the intima allows blood to enter between layers of the wall (Fig. 2-1). Blood pressure then causes the layers of the wall to separate from one another. The serious nature of aneurysms and dissections is due to the weakened vessel wall and the potential for catastrophic events. In the case of an aneurysm, this includes rupture or vascular compromise; dissections can result in the occlusion of the ostia of visceral arteries or progress into the heart and can affect the coronary circulation or lead to tamponade.

ABDOMINAL AORTIC ANEURYSM

Anatomy

The abdominal aorta lies below the diaphragm and above the iliac arteries. Branches include the celiac trunk, superior mesenteric artery, inferior mesenteric artery, renal arteries, and gonadal arteries. Approximately 95% of abdominal aneurysms begin distal to the takeoff of the renal arteries.

Etiology

Ninety-five percent of aneurysms of the abdominal aorta are associated with atherosclerosis. Other causes include trauma, infection, syphilis, and Marfan's syndrome. Protease activity in the vessel wall is commonly increased.

Epidemiology

Abdominal aortic aneurysms are responsible for 15,000 deaths per year. The incidence is approximately 0.05%, but in selected high-risk populations, the incidence increases to 5%. Men are affected ten times more frequently than women, with an age of onset usually between 50 and 70. Risk factors include atherosclerosis, hypertension, hypercholesterolemia, smoking, and obesity. The disease is associated with peripheral vascular disease, heart disease, and carotid artery disease.

History

Most aneurysms are asymptomatic. Pain usually signifies a change in the aneurysm—commonly enlargement, rupture, or compromise of vascular supply—and should therefore be considered an ominous symptom. Pain may occur in the abdomen, back, or flank. The legs could be involved if the aneurysm includes the iliac arteries or if an embolic event occurs. The pain is usually sudden in onset and does not remit.

Physical Examination

Abdominal examination may reveal a pulsatile abdominal mass. Enlargement, rupture, or compromise of vascular supply may manifest by tenderness, hypotension, tachycardia, or a change in the location or intensity of pain. In addition, the lower extremities may have pallor, cool temperature, or pulses that are diminished or unequal.

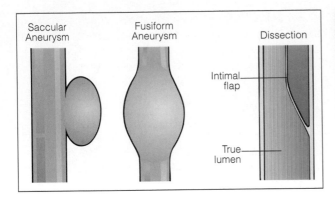

Figure 2-1 • Aneurysms and dissections.

■ TABLE 2-1 Ankle-Brachial Index (ABI)	
Aneurysm Size	Risk of Rupture per Year
Less than 5 cm	4%
5–7 cm	7%
Greater than 7 cm	19%

Diagnostic Evaluation

Ultrasound is an accurate, noninvasive way to assess the size of the aneurysm and the presence of clot within the arterial lumen. Computed tomography (CT) or magnetic resonance imaging (MRI) provides anatomic detail and precise localization of the aneurysm. An aortogram may be helpful in planning surgical intervention to demonstrate involvement of other vessels, specifically the renal, mesenteric, and iliac arteries.

Treatment

If the patient is asymptomatic, workup can proceed electively. Treatment of asymptomatic abdominal aortic aneurysms depends on the size of the lesion, which is directly proportional to its propensity to grow, leak, or rupture. Aneurysms smaller than 4 cm are unlikely to rupture, and medical management with antihypertensives, preferably beta-blockers, is advocated. When the aneurysm reaches approximately 4 to 5 cm, two options are available: early operation or close follow-up. A recent randomized trial suggests that mortality is the same in both options. When the aneurysm reaches 5 cm, the incidence of rupture is greater than 25% at 5 years, and repair is recommended, unless the patient is at prohibitive operative risk. Table 2-1 contains rupture rates per year based on aneurysm size. Treatment options have recently expanded with the advent of stent grafts that can be placed through the femoral artery. In selected patients, these stents carry less morbidity than traditional operative repair, but long-term data are not available. Concerns include stent migration and leaks around the prosthesis. Stent grafts are being used more frequently as experience with them increases. Technologic advances allow placing fenestrated stents with orifices for visceral vessels.

Any patient presenting on physical examination with symptoms that suggest a catastrophic aortic event should undergo emergent diagnostic workup or intervention. Once the diagnosis of ruptured or leaking abdominal aortic aneurysm is determined, arrangements should be made for fluid resuscitation and immediate operative intervention.

Repair of Abdominal Aortic Aneurysm: The Operation

Consistent with the size of the operation, preoperative preparation includes large-bore intravenous lines, central monitoring, and intravenous antibiotics. Blood, either autologous or crossmatched, should be available. Abdominal aortic aneurysms can be approached via either a midline incision or an oblique incision over the 11th intercostal space. Using a midline incision requires mobilization of the small bowel to the patient's right. Incision of the posterior peritoneum to the left of the aorta allows exposure of the entire aorta. The oblique incision is reserved for a retroperitoneal approach, in which the entire contents of the peritoneal cavity are mobilized to the right, allowing exposure of the aorta. Proximal and distal control around the aneurysm is obtained, and heparin is given prior to clamping. A graft is placed using permanent sutures. If a transabdominal approach is used, the peritoneum is closed over the graft if possible (Fig. 2-2).

THORACIC AORTIC ANEURYSM

Anatomy

The thoracic aorta lies between the heart and the diaphragm. It gives rise to the brachiocephalic, left

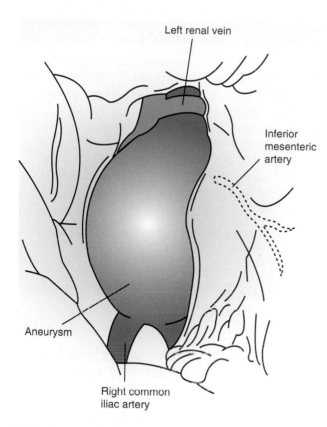

Figure 2-2 • Repair of abdominal aortic aneurysm.
Adapted from Zollinger RM Jr., Zollinger RM Sr. *Zollinger's Atlas of Surgical Operations.* 7th ed. New York, NY: McGraw-Hill; 1993:287.

common carotid, left subclavian, bronchial, esophageal, and intercostal arteries.

Etiology

Thoracic aortic aneurysms are caused by cystic medial necrosis, atherosclerosis, or, less common, trauma, dissection, or infection.

Epidemiology

Males are affected three times as often as females. Risk factors include atherosclerosis, smoking, hypertension, and family history.

History

Most aneurysms are asymptomatic. Rupture usually presents with chest pain or pressure. Expansion of the aneurysm can compress the trachea, leading to cough,

or erode into the trachea or bronchus, causing massive hemoptysis. An aneurysm close to the aortic valve can cause dilation of the annulus, resulting in aortic valve insufficiency and chest pain, dyspnea, or syncope.

Physical Examination

Hypotension and tachycardia may be present. If the aneurysm involves the aortic annulus, it can lead to aortic regurgitation and congestive heart failure. Pulse examination could be abnormal if distal embolization occurs.

Diagnostic Evaluation

Chest radiography may show a widened thoracic aorta. Electrocardiography may demonstrate myocardial ischemia, especially if the aneurysm compromises the coronary supply. In the asymptomatic patient with a thoracic aneurysm, CT or echocardiography is helpful in establishing the diagnosis. Echocardiography can also determine the extent of involvement of the aortic valve and possible cardiac tamponade. Aortography may be useful for planning operative intervention, because it defines the aneurysm's relation to a number of critical structures.

Treatment

As with abdominal aortic aneurysms, operative repair should be considered when the maximum diameter approaches 5 cm. Symptomatic presentation is an indication for immediate operative intervention. As with abdominal aortic aneurysms, the indications for stent grafts for thoracic aortic aneurysms are being carefully evaluated.

AORTIC DISSECTION

Pathogenesis

Dissections can be due to hypertension, trauma, Marfan syndrome, or aortic coarctation.

Epidemiology

Aortic dissections are more common than either thoracic or abdominal aneurysms. Incidence increases with age, and males are more commonly affected than females.

History

Patients usually complain of the immediate onset of severe pain, often described as tearing, usually in the chest, back, or abdomen. Nausea or light-headedness may also be present.

Physical Examination

Patients may be hypotensive. Rales on chest auscultation or a new murmur suggest that the dissection continues retrograde into the aortic root. Peripheral pulses are diminished if distal blood flow is compromised. If the dissection continues into the visceral arteries, compromise of mesenteric vessels can produce abdominal pain, compromise of renal arteries can cause oliguria, and compromise of spinal blood supply can produce neurologic deficits.

Diagnostic Evaluation

A chest radiograph may show a widened mediastinum. CT may show the dissection or clot in the arterial lumen. Diagnosis can be made with transesophageal ultrasound, MRI, or aortogram. Dissections are classified according to the DeBakey classification: Type I involve both the ascending and the descending aorta, type II involve only the ascending aorta, and type III involve only the descending aorta.

Treatment

Dissection of the ascending thoracic aorta usually requires surgery, because of the potential for retrograde progression into the aortic root and subsequent compromise of the coronary circulation or tamponade from rupture into the pericardium. Eighty percent of patients with involvement of the ascending aorta die without treatment. Antihypertensive therapy is used preoperatively in an attempt to halt the progression of the dissection.

In contrast, dissections limited to the descending aorta are best managed medically, with antihypertensives, including sodium nitroprusside and beta blockade. Invasive monitoring with fluid resuscitation should be instituted immediately. Surgery is reserved for lesions that progress or cause distal ischemia. Stent grafts have been shown to be safe in selected patients. Determination of who should receive a stent graft is being studied.

🔑 2-1 KEY POINTS

1. Aneurysms and dissections can be rapidly fatal.
2. Repair via open operation or stent graft should be considered for asymptomatic aneurysms greater than 4 or 5 cm.
3. Symptomatic aneurysms or dissections require emergency diagnosis and treatment.
4. Dissections that involve the ascending aorta usually require surgery, whereas dissections that involve the descending aorta are best managed medically.

CAROTID ARTERY DISEASE

ANATOMY

The common carotid artery on the right arises from the brachiocephalic artery, and on the left, from the aorta. The common carotid then bifurcates into internal and external branches. The internal carotid gives off the ophthalmic artery before continuing to the circle of Willis to supply the brain.

PATHOGENESIS

Symptoms are the result of atherosclerosis. Mechanisms of morbidity include plaque rupture, ulceration, hemorrhage, thrombosis, and low flow states. Because of the rich collateralization of the cerebral circulation through the circle of Willis, thrombosis and low flow states may be asymptomatic.

EPIDEMIOLOGY

Atherosclerotic occlusive disease of the carotid artery is a major cause of stroke. In the United States, 400,000 people are hospitalized for stroke each year, and cerebrovascular events are the third most common cause of death. The incidence of stroke increases with age. Other risk factors include hypertension, diabetes, smoking, and hypercholesterolemia. Markers for carotid disease include evidence of other atherosclerotic disease and prior neurologic events.

HISTORY

Patients often relate previous neurologic events, including focal motor deficits, weakness, clumsiness, and expressive or cognitive aphasia. These could occur as a transient ischemic attack (TIA), which resolves in 24 hours; a reversible ischemic neurologic deficit, which resolves in greater than 24 hours; or a fixed neurologic deficit. One characteristic presentation for carotid disease is amaurosis fugax, or transient monocular blindness, usually described as a shade being pulled down in front of the patient's eye. This is due to occlusion of a branch of the ophthalmic artery.

PHYSICAL EXAMINATION

Patients may exhibit a fixed neurologic deficit. Hollenhorst plaques on retinal examination are evidence of previous emboli. A carotid bruit is evidence of turbulence in carotid blood flow, but the presence of a bruit does not unequivocally translate into a hemodynamically significant lesion, and the absence of a bruit does not unequivocally indicate the absence of significant disease.

DIAGNOSTIC EVALUATION

Carotid duplex scanning is both sensitive and specific for carotid disease. Conventional or magnetic resonance angiography is more accurate for assessing the degree of stenosis.

TREATMENT

Treatment depends on the history, degree of stenosis, and characteristics of the plaque. Antiplatelet therapy with aspirin is effective in preventing neurologic events. When dealing with an acute event, heparin should be considered after head CT determines that the event is not hemorrhagic. Indications for carotid endarterectomy are controversial. Results of two large randomized controlled trials—the Asymptomatic Carotid Atherosclerosis Study (ACAS) and the North American Symptomatic Carotid Endarterectomy Trial (NASCET)—suggest surgery is best reserved for the following patients: those with greater than 75% stenosis, those with 70% stenosis and symptoms, those with bilateral disease and symptoms, or those with greater than 50% stenosis and recurring TIAs despite aspirin therapy. The role of stenting is controversial. Despite the SAPPHIRE trial, which suggested stenting is not inferior to endarterectomy in high-risk patients, there were problems with the study design, and the procedure is still being evaluated as an alternative to open surgery, which has very low morbidity and mortality in large centers.

CAROTID ENDARTERECTOMY: THE OPERATION

Perioperative monitoring is surgeon dependent. Techniques include keeping the patient awake through the procedure, using local or regional anesthesia, using continuous electroencephalogram (EEG) monitoring, or using no monitoring at all. Administration of intravenous antibiotics, usually a first generation cephalosporin, precedes the incision. After site verification, the neck is extended, and an incision is made over the anterior border of the sternocleidomastoid muscle. Dissection continues through the platysma and along the sternocleidomastoid. Ligation of the facial vein allows complete exposure of the carotid, which lies just medial to the jugular vein. Care is taken not to injure the hypoglossal nerve at the superior aspect of the dissection or the spinal accessory nerve (Fig. 2-3). Proximal and distal control of the carotid is obtained, the patient is heparinized, and the artery is opened after clamps are applied. Use of a stent may provide cerebral protection. Plaque is carefully dissected out of the artery, and the artery is usually closed with a patch.

🔑 2-2 KEY POINTS

1. Carotid artery disease is a major cause of stroke in the United States.
2. Indications for operation include 75% stenosis, 70% stenosis and symptoms, bilateral disease and symptoms, or greater than 50% stenosis and recurring transient ischemic attacks despite aspirin therapy.
3. Stenting is an option for selected patients.

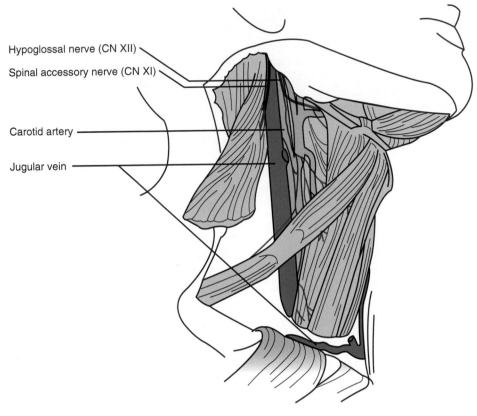

Hypoglossal nerve (CN XII)

Spinal accessory nerve (CN XI)

Carotid artery

Jugular vein

Figure 2-3 • Carotid endarterectomy: pertinent anatomical structures.

ACUTE AND CHRONIC MESENTERIC VASCULAR DISEASE

ANATOMY

Acute and chronic mesenteric vascular disease includes disease of the celiac axis, which is the arterial supply to the liver, spleen, pancreas, and stomach; the superior mesenteric artery, which supplies the pancreas, small bowel, and proximal colon; and inferior mesenteric artery, which supplies the distal colon and rectum. In addition, thrombosis of the superior mesenteric vein can cause visceral ischemia.

PATHOGENESIS

Acute ischemia is caused by acute embolization, acute thrombosis, nonocclusive ischemia, and mesenteric vein thrombosis. Embolization is associated with atherosclerotic disease or mural cardiac thrombus. Acute thrombosis is associated with atherosclerosis and hypercoagulable states. Vasopressor agents can produce acute ischemia. Chronic ischemia usually requires severe atherosclerotic disease in at least two major arterial trunks among the superior and inferior mesenteric arteries and the celiac axis, because of the extensive collateralization.

EPIDEMIOLOGY

The incidence of acute mesenteric ischemia is estimated at 1 in 1,000 hospital admissions, and mortality is greater than 50%. Prevalence of chronic ischemia increases with age, and risk factors include hypertension, smoking, hypercholesterolemia, and diabetes.

HISTORY

Patients with acute ischemia may have a history of previous embolic events, atrial fibrillation, or congestive failure. Abdominal pain is usually sudden in onset and is severe, with diarrhea or vomiting. History in chronic mesenteric ischemia usually reveals crampy abdominal pain after eating. This results in decreased oral intake and weight loss. Nausea, vomiting, constipation, or diarrhea may occur. The disease can be mistaken for malignant disease or cholelithiasis.

PHYSICAL EXAMINATION

In episodes of acute ischemia, the classic finding is "pain out of proportion to physical examination." The abdomen may be distended. Rectal examination often reveals guaiac-positive stool. Atrial fibrillation may be present. Physical findings in chronic ischemia include abdominal bruits, guaiac-positive stool, and evidence of peripheral vascular disease or coronary artery disease.

DIAGNOSTIC EVALUATION

In acute ischemia, there could be an elevated white blood cell count, metabolic acidosis, or an elevated hematocrit as fluid is sequestered in the infarcting bowel. Abdominal radiographs are often normal in the early phase of the disease, but as the intestine becomes edematous, "thumbprinting" of the bowel wall occurs. Evaluation in chronic ischemia includes selective visceral angiography to identify the site of the lesion.

TREATMENT

Once the diagnosis of acute ischemia is made, laparotomy with examination and resection of any infarcted bowel should be considered. In selected cases, angiography can be therapeutic, as well as diagnostic, with catheter-based therapies. Aggressive surgical intervention should not be delayed if there is a suspicion of dead bowel. Despite aggressive intervention, mortality is extremely high. For chronic ischemia, angiography can define the lesion and allow consideration of surgical options. Acute mesenteric vein thrombosis is treated with anticoagulation and laparotomy if necrotic bowel is suspected.

🔑 2-3 KEY POINTS

1. Patients with acute mesenteric ischemia present with "pain out of proportion to examination," and a mechanism for embolic disease is usually present.
2. Chronic mesenteric ischemia results in weight loss and abdominal pain and is frequently mistaken for malignant disease.

PERIPHERAL VASCULAR DISEASE

ANATOMY

Lesions may occur in the iliac, common and superficial femoral, popliteal, peroneal, anterior tibial, and posterior tibial arteries. In general, of the three vessels that supply the distal ankle and foot, a single direct arterial supply is adequate to prevent limb loss and rest pain.

PATHOGENESIS

In *acute disease*, the most common cause is an embolus that causes a sudden decrease in blood flow. The most common sources are the aorta and the heart. Rarer causes include acute arterial thrombosis, acute venous thrombosis, and arterial spasm. In *chronic disease*, progressive atherosclerotic disease causes narrowing of the arterial lumen and decreased blood flow. Pain occurs as decreased blood flow is unable to meet the metabolic and waste-removal demand of the tissue.

EPIDEMIOLOGY

Acute disease occurs in patients with cardiac thrombus, atrial fibrillation, or atherosclerosis. Risk factors for chronic disease include atherosclerosis, smoking, diabetes, hypertension, and advanced age.

HISTORY

Acute ischemia causes sudden and severe lower extremity pain and paresthesias. Patients with chronic ischemia typically present with claudication, defined as reproducible pain on exercise relieved by rest. The site of claudication provides a clue to the level of disease. Buttock claudication usually indicates aortoiliac disease, whereas calf claudication suggests femoral atherosclerosis. Pain at rest is indicative of severe disease and a threatened limb. Slow or nonhealing ulcers may be present.

PHYSICAL EXAMINATION

In acute disease, the patient may exhibit pulselessness, pallor, and poikilothermia (coolness). Taken together with pain and paresthesia, these form the five *p*'s of

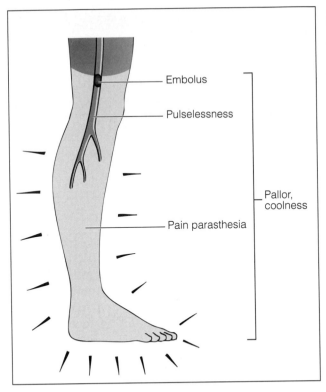

Embolus

Pulselessness

Pallor, coolness

Pain parasthesia

Figure 2-4 • Signs and symptoms of acute embolus.

acute vascular compromise (Fig. 2-4). In chronic disease, the lower extremity may reveal loss of hair, pallor on elevation, rubor on placing the extremity in a dependent position, wasting of musculature, thick nails, and thin skin. The extremity may be cool to the touch, and pulses may be diminished or absent. Ulcers or frank necrosis may be present.

DIAGNOSTIC EVALUATION

Angiography is necessary in cases of acute ischemia to identify the lesion. Evaluation for chronic ischemia

includes Doppler flow measurement of distal pulses. The normal signal is triphasic; as disease progresses, the signal becomes biphasic, monophasic, and then absent. Ankle-brachial indices of less than 0.5 are indicative of significant disease (Table 2-1). Arteriography is the gold standard for defining the level and extent of disease and for planning surgery.

TREATMENT

Acute ischemic embolus can be treated with heparin, thrombolysis, or embolectomy. For chronic ischemia, patients with claudication have a low rate of limb loss, and initial therapy is based on smoking cessation and a graded exercise program. Success rates with nonoperative therapy are good. In patients with disabling claudication, threatened limbs, nonhealing ulcers, or gangrene, angioplasty or revascularization should be considered (Table 2-2). It is always prudent to consider amputation in selected patients with long-standing acute ischemia or chronic ischemia, though this decision is often a difficult one and requires experience and careful discussions with the patient.

PERIPHERAL BYPASS: THE OPERATION

Patients usually have concurrent coronary artery disease, and preoperative evaluation and intraoperative beta blockade should be considered. The entire leg is usually prepped. Intravenous antibiotics are often a first-generation cephalosporin, and central monitoring should be considered. The most common techniques for anesthesia include general and regional. If the proximal vessels are open, inflow is usually from the femoral artery, which is dissected via an infrainguinal incision directly over the artery. If the target is the popliteal, it is isolated via an incision over the

■ **TABLE 2-2** Progression of Peripheral Vascular Disease			
	Claudication	**Rest Pain**	**Gangrene**
Blood flow	Decreased	Markedly decreased	Minimal
ABI	~0.5	0.3–0.5	<0.3
Treatment	Smoking cessation	Revascularization	Amputation
	Graded exercise	Angioplasty	Revascularization
			Angioplasty

medial aspect of the knee, at the level where the out-flow will be targeted. If the target is the dorsalis pedis, tibialis anterior, or peroneal, the incision is made directly over the target. Above-knee popliteal reconstruction can be accomplished with synthetic grafts, but infrapopliteal reconstructions should use either in situ or reversed saphenous vein.

🔑 2-4 KEY POINTS

1. Acute peripheral embolus is marked by the five *p*'s.
2. Symptoms of chronic peripheral vascular disease usually follow a well-defined progression.
3. Operation should be considered only in patients with severe chronic peripheral vascular disease.

References

Chaturvedi S, Bruno A, Feasby T, Holloway R, Benavente O, Cohen SN, et al. Carotid endarterectomy—An evidence-based review: report of the Therapeutics and Technology Assessment Subcommittee of the American Academy of Neurology. *Neurology.* 2005;65(6):794–801.

Norton JA, Barie PS, Bollinger RR, et al., eds. *Surgery: Basic Science and Clinical Evidence.* New York, NY: Springer; 2001.

Sakalihasan N, Limet R, Defawe OD. Abdominal aortic aneurysm. *Lancet.* 2005;365(9470):1577–1589.

Breast

ANATOMY AND PHYSIOLOGY

The breast is composed of glandular tissue ventral to the pectoralis major muscle. Support is provided by Cooper's ligaments. The functional units are lobules that contain terminal ducts, where milk is produced, and ductules and ducts that convey the milk to the nipple. The lymphatic drainage travels through axillary, mammary, and central nodes. Nodes are characterized based on their relation to the pectoralis minor. Level 1 nodes are lateral to the muscle, level 2 nodes are beneath it, and level 3 nodes are medial to it. In the axilla lie the thoracodorsal nerve, which provides motor function to the latissimus dorsi, and the long thoracic nerve, which provides motor function to the serratus anterior (Fig. 3-1). Damage to the thoracodorsal or long thoracic nerves during dissection leads to weakness in shoulder abduction or a winged scapula, respectively.

PATHOLOGY

Benign breast lesions include simple cysts, fibroadenomas, papillomas, and "fibrocystic disease," a group of findings that include firm nodular lesions, cysts, and epithelial hyperplasia. Tumors with low malignant potential include phyllodes tumors. The most common malignant lesions are lobular and ductal carcinoma. These occur in noninvasive or in situ forms that do not penetrate the basement membrane and in invasive forms that do. Inflammatory breast cancer is characterized by tumor invasion of lymphatic channels. Paget's disease occurs when tumor cells invade the epidermal layer of the skin.

EPIDEMIOLOGY

Breast cancer is the second leading cause of cancer deaths among women. It is estimated that between 1 in 9 and 1 in 11 women will be diagnosed with breast cancer during their lifetimes. Significant risk factors include age (breast cancer before age 30 is rare), history of breast cancer in a first-degree relative (two to three times normal risk; higher if the relative had premenopausal cancer), atypical hyperplasia diagnosed on previous biopsy (four times normal risk), personal history of breast cancer, and lobular carcinoma in situ (LCIS). Risk factors that are less important include early menarche and late menopause. Ductal carcinoma is the most common breast malignancy. Simple cysts, fibroadenomas, fibrocystic change, and papillomas are not associated with increased risk of breast cancer. Fibroadenoma is the most common tumor in young women. Intraductal papilloma is the most common cause of bloody nipple discharge.

HISTORY

Women with breast cancer may relate the discovery of a new mass. Malignant lesions are usually not cyclic with menses, whereas simple cysts are. Masses that increase in size are cause for concern. Patients with cancer may have constitutional symptoms, including weight loss, nausea, and malaise. Bone pain is an ominous symptom that may signify skeletal metastases. Intraductal papilloma may present with nipple discharge. Patients with inflammatory cancer may describe warmth or tenderness at the site.

PHYSICAL EXAMINATION

Fibroadenomas are usually well circumscribed and mobile. Breast asymmetry, dimpling or retractions, and excoriation or edema of the skin are extremely sensitive for malignancy. Characteristics of malignancy on palpation include firmness and indistinct border

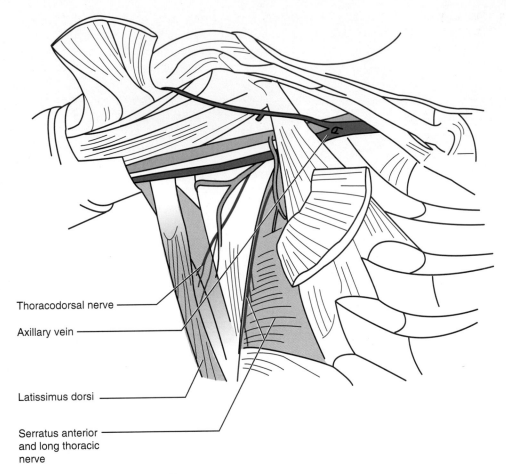

Thoracodorsal nerve

Axillary vein

Latissimus dorsi

Serratus anterior
and long thoracic
nerve

Figure 3-1 • Anatomy of the axilla.

Lymphadenopathy may be present, and there may be bloody discharge. Inflammatory cancer may display erythema and skin excoriation, termed *peau d'orange*. Paget disease may present with nipple or areolar excoriation. Phyllodes tumors usually present as a painless mass.

DIAGNOSTIC EVALUATION

Screening mammography has been shown by a number of studies to decrease mortality from breast cancer. Though routine use has been extremely controversial, most national organizations recommend its use as a screening tool. The current recommendations from the American Cancer Society are for a baseline mammogram between the ages of 35 and 39, every to 2 years between the ages of 40 and 50, and yearly

after age 50. Patients with a family history of breast cancer are often advised to begin screening earlier, but it is not clear that this practice has benefits in terms of outcomes. Characteristics on a mammogram that are suspicious for malignancy include densities with irregular margins, spiculated lesions, microcalcifications, or rodlike or branching patterns. Any changes from a previous mammogram should be viewed with concern, and any suspicious mass should be considered for biopsy. Needle-directed biopsy is useful for nonpalpable mammographic abnormalities. This technique uses mammographic guidance to place a needle at the lesion, which the surgeon later uses to locate it. Palpable masses should be considered for fine-needle aspiration. Cancer is unlikely if all of the following criteria are met: The mass completely disappears after aspiration, it does not return, and the fluid is hemoccult-negative. Aspirate should be sent for cytology, which has a sensitivity of 70% to 90%, depending on the cytologist and the surgeon. If any of these criteria are not met, biopsy should be performed.

TREATMENT

Surgical Procedures—Lumpectomy involves removal of the lesion with negative margins. Mastectomy is removal of all breast tissue on the affected side. Axillary node dissection involves removal of all level I and II nodes. Modified radical mastectomy combines mastectomy with axillary node dissection. Sentinel node biopsy is a relatively new procedure that merits particular attention. It is replacing complete axillary node dissection to evaluate the axilla in patients with early stage disease. This procedure consists of injecting a vital blue dye or radioactive sulfur colloid, or both, around the tumor. The surgeon then waits 5 minutes in the case of the dye and a few hours in the case of the colloid and dissects the axilla, removing only a few nodes that are either stained blue or radioactive. The principle behind this is that the first nodes that drain the dye are the ones most likely to first drain the tumor. Multiple studies demonstrate decreased morbidity compared to a full axillary node dissection, and in experienced hands, the procedure is close to 100% accurate in correctly describing the presence or absence of tumor in the axilla. In the presence of a positive sentinel node, complete axillary dissection can be performed at the same setting or later.

Ductal Carcinoma in Situ (DCIS)—DCIS is a premalignant lesion. There are two major therapeutic options. The first is local excision with negative margins followed by radiation. Radiation may not be necessary in patients with small, low-grade lesions. The second option is mastectomy without radiation. This is generally preferred if the lesion is large, if negative margins are unable to be obtained, or the patient prefers this approach. Long-term outcomes are similar between the two options, with survival approaching 100%.

Lobular Carcinoma in Situ (LCIS)—LCIS is best considered a condition rather than a lesion. Women with LCIS carry an increased risk of breast cancer but the cancer can occur in either breast and is unrelated to the lesion biopsied. For this reason, local excision is not recommended. There are two treatment options. The first is careful follow-up including physical exams and mammography. The next option is thought extreme by some and consists of bilateral prophylactic mastectomy. This should only be performed in selected cases, for example if follow-up is not possible, or if there is an extremely strong family history of aggressive breast cancer.

Stage I or II breast cancer (Tables 3-1 and 3-2)—Treatment for these lesions are based on surgical removal of the tumor with negative margins and assessment of the regional lymph nodes. Surgical options are lumpectomy or mastectomy. Relative indications that favor mastectomy include multiple tumors, prior radiation, large lesions, and positive lumpectomy margins. If mastectomy is chosen, radiation should be added as it decreases local recurrence rates. Long-term survival is the same in both gropus. Assessment of regional lymph nodes is generally performed by sentinel node biopsy,

■ TABLE 3-1 TNM Staging for Breast Cancer	
Stage	**Description**
Tumor	
TX	Primary tumor not assessable
T0	No evidence of primary tumor
Tis	Carcinoma in situ
T1	Tumor 2 cm or less in greatest dimension
T2	Tumor more than 2 cm but not more than 5 cm in greatest dimension
T3	Tumor more than 5 cm in greatest dimension
T4	Tumor of any size with direct extension into chest wall (not including pectoral muscles) or skin edema or skin ulceration or satellite skin nodules confined to the same breast or inflammatory carcinoma
Regional lymph nodes	
NX	Regional lymph nodes not assessable
N0	No regional lymph node involvement
N1	Metastasis to movable ipsilateral axillary lymph node(s)
N2	Metastasis to ipsilateral axillary lymph node(s) fixed to one another or to other structures
N3	Metastasis to ipsilateral internal mammary lymph nodes
Distant metastasis	
MX	Presence of distant metastasis cannot be assessed
M0	No distant metastasis
M1	Distant metastasis present (including ipsilateral supraclavicular lymph nodes)

TNM, tumor, nodes, metastases.

TABLE 3-2 AJCC Classification for Breast Cancer Based on TNM Criteria

Stage	Tumor	Nodes	Metastases
0	Tis	N0	M0
I	T1	N0	M0
IIA	T0, 1	N1	M0
	T2	N0	M0
IIB	T2	N1	M0
	T3	N0	M0
IIIA	T0, 1, 2	N2	M0
	T3	N1, 2	M0
IIIB	T4	N1, 2	M0
	Any T	N3	M0
IV	Any T	Any N	M1

AJCC, American Joint Committee on Cancer; TNM, tumor, nodes, metastases.
AJCC Cancer Staging manual, Sixth Edition. (2002) published by Springer-Verlag New York

though if the original lesion is greater than 5 cm, complete axillary node dissection may be preferable.

Chemotherapy and radiation are offered but in general are being used more for early-stage lesions in the absence of rigorous clinical data.

Stage III or IV disease (see Tables 3-1 and 3-2)—Surgical resection for local control and radiation or chemotherapy is beneficial (see Table 3-3). Because surgery treats only the local manifestations of a disseminated disease, resection should not be the basis of treatment.

Endocrine therapy is an effective, low risk treatment for certain types of breast cancers. Tumors that express the estrogen receptor have a 30% probability of responding to endocrine therapy. If the tumor also expresses the progesterone receptor the probability increaes to 70%. Newer aromatase inhibitors that prevent the production of estrone and estradiol are generally superior to tamoxifen.

Chemotherapeutic options are highly individualized. Common regimens include CMF (cyclophosphamide, methotrexate, and 5-fluorouracil), AC (doxorubicin, cyclophosphamide), and tamoxifen. Because

of the relatively serious side effect of the first two regimens, treatment choices are based on the extent of the tumor and the patient's general medical condition.

Newer agents including Herceptin, gemcitabine, capecitabine, navelbine, and etoposide may be useful in previously treated patients and are being evaluated as adjuvant therapy.

PROGNOSIS

Patients with stage I disease have an approximately 80% 5-year disease-free survival rate, stage II disease carries a 60% 5-year disease-free survival rate, and stage III disease portends only a 20% 5-year disease-free survival rate. Patients with stage IV disease have minimal long-term survival. The presence of estrogen and progesterone receptors independently improves survival rates.

3-1 KEY POINTS

1. Breast cancer is the second leading cause of cancer deaths among women.
2. Significant risk factors include age, family or personal history, atypical hyperplasia on biopsy, and lobular carcinoma in situ.
3. Mammography decreases mortality. Current recommendations are for a baseline mammogram between 35 and 39 years of age and then mammograms every 1 to 2 years between the ages of 40 and 50 and every year thereafter.
4. A palpable abnormality should not be dismissed because of a normal mammogram, and a mammographic abnormality should not be dismissed because the mass is not palpable.
5. Treatment options for ductal carcinoma in situ include mastectomy or lumpectomy and radiation.
6. Surgical options for invasive cancer include modified radical mastectomy or lumpectomy with axillary node dissection and radiation. Sentinel node biopsy will probably replace axillary dissection as the treatment of choice in the near future.

References

Bafaloukos D. Neo-adjuvant therapy in breast cancer. *Ann Oncol.* 2005;16(suppl 2):ii, 174–181.

Burak WE Jr., Agnese DM, Povoski SP. Advances in the surgical management of early stage invasive breast cancer. *Curr Probl Surg.* 2004;41(11): 882–935.

Mamounas EP. NSABP breast cancer clinical trials: recent results and future directions. *Clin Med Res.* 2003;1(4):309–326.

Norton JA, Barie PS, Bollinger RR, et al., eds. *Surgery: Basic Science and Clinical Evidence.* New York, NY: Springer; 2001.

ANATOMY AND PHYSIOLOGY

The colon begins at the ileocecal valve and extends to the anal canal. Its primary function is the reabsorption of water and sodium, secretion of potassium and bicarbonate, and storage of fecal material. The ascending and descending colon are fixed in a retroperitoneal location, whereas the transverse and sigmoid colon are intraperitoneal. Arterial supply to the cecum, ascending colon, and proximal to the midtransverse colon is from the superior mesenteric artery (SMA) by way of the ileocolic, right colic, and middle colic arteries. The remainder of the colon is supplied by the inferior mesenteric artery (IMA) by way of the left colic, sigmoid, and superior hemorrhoidal arteries and the middle and inferior hemorrhoidal arteries that arise from the internal iliac artery. The long anastomosis between the SMA and IMA is called the *anastomosis of Riolan,* and the arcades in proximity to the mesenteric border of the colon are referred to as the *marginal artery of Drummond* (Fig. 4-1). Venous drainage from the colon includes the superior and inferior mesenteric veins (SMV and IMV, respectively). The IMV joins the splenic vein, which joins the SMV to form the portal vein. In this way, mesenteric blood flow enters the liver, where it is detoxified before entering the central circulation. Lymphatic drainage follows the arteries and veins.

ULCERATIVE COLITIS

Ulcerative colitis is an inflammatory disease of the colon with unknown etiology. It almost always involves the rectum and extends backward toward the cecum to varying degrees.

PATHOLOGY

Inflammation is confined to the mucosa and submucosa. Superficial ulcers, thickened mucosa, crypt abscesses, and pseudopolyps may also be present.

EPIDEMIOLOGY

The incidence is 6 per 100,000. The disease commonly presents in the third or fourth decade. It is more common in developed countries, especially among Caucasians and the Jewish population. There is no predilection for sex. Approximately 20% of patients have first-degree relatives who are affected. Linkage analysis has identified an association with human leukocyte antigens (HLA) AW24 and BW25.

HISTORY

Patients commonly complain of bloody diarrhea, fever, abdominal pain, and weight loss. Multiple attacks are common. A number of diseases are associated with ulcerative colitis, including sclerosing cholangitis in 1% of patients, as well as arthritis, iritis, cholangitis, aphthous ulcers, and ankylosing spondylosis. These diseases may be part of the initial presentation.

PHYSICAL EXAMINATION

Abdominal pain is common. Rectal tenderness may occur with rectal fissures. The disease may present with abdominal distention as evidence of massive colonic distention, a situation known as toxic megacolon. This may progress to frank perforation with signs of peritonitis.

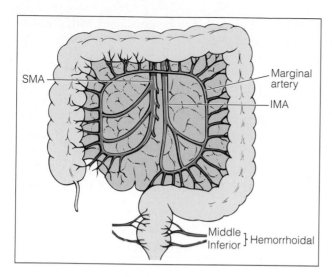

Figure 4-1 • Arterial supply of the colon. SMA, superior mesenteric artery; IMA, inferior mesenteric artery.

DIAGNOSTIC EVALUATION

Colonoscopy may demonstrate thickened, friable mucosa. Fissures and pseudopolyps, if present, almost always involve the rectum and varying portions of the colon. Biopsy shows ulceration limited to the mucosa and submucosa; crypt abscesses may be present. Barium enema may reveal a stovepipe colon with smooth edges and ulcers.

COMPLICATIONS

Perforation or obstruction may develop from stricture. Hemorrhage or toxic megacolon is uncommon but may be life-threatening. Colon cancer occurs frequently, with a risk of approximately 10% within 20 years.

TREATMENT

Initial therapy is medical, with fluid administration, electrolyte correction, and parenteral nutrition if necessary. Steroids, other immunosuppressives, and sulfasalazine are all effective. Topical mesalamine, in the form of enemas, is effective for mild and moderate disease. Newer immunosuppressive agents—including infliximab, a monoclonal antibody against tumor necrosis factor—may be useful. Indications for surgery include colonic obstruction, massive blood loss, failure of medical therapy, toxic megacolon, and cancer. The recommendation of prophylactic colectomy for these patients is being reconsidered based on recent data

that suggest the incidence of cancer is not as high as once thought. With sphincter-sparing operations, continence and bowel movements can be preserved.

🔑 4-1 KEY POINTS

1. Ulcerative colitis presents with bloody diarrhea and abdominal pain. Pathologic changes are limited to the mucosa and submucosa.
2. Patients with ulcerative colitis have a significant risk of colon cancer.
3. Surgery for ulcerative colitis is used for intractable bleeding, obstruction, failure of medical therapy, toxic megacolon, and risk of cancer.

DIVERTICULOSIS

Diverticulosis refers to the presence of diverticula, outpouchings of the colon wall that occur at points where the arterial supply penetrates the bowel wall. These are false diverticula because not all layers of the bowel wall are included. Most diverticula occur in the sigmoid colon. Diverticulosis is the most common cause of lower gastrointestinal hemorrhage, usually from the right colon. Of people with diverticulosis, 15% will have a significant episode of bleeding.

EPIDEMIOLOGY

Diverticular disease is common in developed nations and is likely related to low-fiber diets. Men and women are equally affected, and the prevalence increases dramatically with age. Approximately one third of the population has diverticular disease, but this number increases to more than half of those over age 80.

HISTORY

Patients usually present with bleeding from the rectum without other complaints. They may have had previous episodes of bleeding or crampy abdominal pain, commonly in the left lower quadrant.

DIAGNOSTIC EVALUATION

For patients who stop bleeding spontaneously, elective colonoscopy should be performed to determine the etiology of the bleeding. If bleeding continues, diagnostic and therapeutic modalities include radioisotope bleeding scans, which have variable success rates, and mesenteric angiography, which has an excellent success rate in the presence of active bleeding.

TREATMENT

Asymptomatic individuals require no treatment. In the event of a bleed, 80% will stop spontaneously. Elective segmental or subtotal colectomy is not usually recommended at first episode; however, depending on the ability to accurately determine the site of bleeding, the severity of the initial presentation, and the general status of the patient, it can be offered. Patients with recurrent bleeding are usually offered surgical resection. Active bleeding is treated colonoscopically if the colon can be cleaned. Embolization of the bleeding vessel may be possible using angiography. If these methods fail and no bleeding site is identified, emergent subtotal colectomy is performed, which involves removing most of the colon. If the bleeding site is identified, segmental colectomy can be performed, usually based on the arterial branch feeding the bleeding site.

🔑 4-2 KEY POINTS

1. Diverticulosis is the most common cause of lower gastrointestinal bleeding.
2. Surgical therapy for diverticulosis is recommended for recurrent or intractable bleeding.

DIVERTICULITIS

The narrow neck of the diverticula predisposes it to infection, which occurs either from increased intraluminal pressure or inspissated food particles. Infection leads to localized or free perforation into the abdomen. Diverticulitis most commonly occurs in the sigmoid and is rare in the right colon. Approximately 20% of patients with diverticula experience an episode of diverticulitis. Each attack makes a subsequent attack more likely and increases the risk of complications.

HISTORY

Patients usually present with left lower quadrant pain; right-sided diverticulitis causes right-sided pain but is less common. The pain is usually progressive over a few days and may be associated with diarrhea or constipation.

PHYSICAL EXAMINATION

Abdominal tenderness, usually in the left lower quadrant, is the most common finding. Local peritoneal signs of rebound and guarding may be present. Diffuse rebound tenderness or guarding as evidence of generalized peritonitis suggests free intra-abdominal perforation.

DIAGNOSTIC EVALUATION

The white blood cell count is usually elevated. Radiographs of the abdomen are usually normal. Computed tomography (CT) may demonstrate pericolic fat stranding, bowel wall thickening, or an abscess. Colonoscopy and barium enema should not be performed during an acute episode because of the risk of causing or exacerbating an existing perforation.

COMPLICATIONS

Stricture, perforation, or fistulization with the bladder, skin, vagina, or other portions of the bowel may develop.

TREATMENT

Most episodes of diverticulitis are mild and can be treated on an outpatient basis with broad-spectrum oral antibiotics. Ciprofloxacin and metronidazole (Flagyl) would be an appropriate choice to cover bowel flora. For severe cases or cases in elderly or debilitated patients, hospitalization with bowel rest and broad-spectrum intravenous antibiotics (e.g., ampicillin, levofloxacin, and metronidazole) are required. For patients who do not improve in 48 hours on this regimen, repeated CT with drainage of any abscess cavity may obviate the need for emergency operation. In the event of free perforation or failure of the modalities discussed, surgical drainage with colostomy is required. In addition, surgical resection is indicated in the presence of the complications previously described as well as after a second attack because the risk of subsequent attacks increases; the risk of complications with a second attack is 60%.

4-3 KEY POINTS

1. Patients with diverticulitis usually present with left lower quadrant pain.
2. Surgical therapy for diverticulitis is indicated after a second attack because of the high recurrence and complication rate.

COLONIC NEOPLASMS

Recent evidence suggests that colon cancer follows an orderly progression in which adenomatous polyps undergo malignant transformation over a variable time period. For this reason, these polyps are considered premalignant lesions. Fifty percent of carcinomas have a ras gene mutation, whereas 75% have a p53 gene mutation.

EPIDEMIOLOGY

Colon cancer is the second most common cause of cancer death in the United States. Risk factors include high-fat and low-fiber diets, age, and family history. Ulcerative colitis, Crohn's disease, and Gardner's syndrome all predispose to cancer, and cancer develops in all patients with familial polyposis coli if they are not treated.

PATHOLOGY

Adenomatous polyps are tubular or villous, with some lesions exhibiting features of both. The higher the villous component, the higher the risk of malignancy. As the lesion grows in size, the likelihood of its having undergone malignant transformation increases significantly. Although tubular adenomas under 1 cm contain malignancy in only 1% of cases, lesions greater than 2 cm contain malignancy 25% of the time. For villous adenomas, the numbers are 10% and 50%. Ninety percent of colon cancers are adenocarcinomas, and 20% of these are mucinous, carrying the worst prognosis. Other types include squamous, adenosquamous, lymphoma, sarcoma, and carcinoid.

SCREENING

Screening is aimed at detecting polyps and early malignant lesions. The current screening recommendations from the American Gastroenterological Association divide people into two groups: Average-risk persons have no risk factors. Increased-risk persons have a history of adenomatous polyps or colorectal cancer, first-degree relatives with colorectal cancer or adenomatous polyps, family history of multiple cancers, or a history of inflammatory bowel disease. Screening should begin at age 50 for average-risk patients and age 40 for increased-risk patients. Screening should include a yearly fecal occult blood test, sigmoidoscopy every 3 to 5 years, and colonoscopy or barium enema approximately every 10 years.

STAGING

Staging of colon cancer follows the TNM (tumor, nodes, metastases) classification or Dukes' classification (Table 4-1). TNM classification is as follows: T1: Tumor invades submucosa. T2: Tumor invades muscularis propria. T3: Tumor invades through the muscularis propria into the subserosa or into the pericolic or perirectal tissues. T4: Tumor directly invades other organs or structures or perforates, or both. N0: No regional lymph node metastasis. N1: Metastasis in one to three regional lymph nodes. N2: Metastasis in four or more regional lymph nodes. M0: No distant metastasis. M1: Distant metastasis present. Stage 1 tumors are T1, N0, M0 or T2, N0, M0. Stage 2 tumors are T3, N0, M0 or T4, N0, M0. Stage 3 tumors are any T, N1 or N2, M0. Stage 4 tumors are M1. Dukes' A lesions are limited to the mucosa without lymph node involvement. B lesions have no lymph node involvement. B1 lesions involve the muscularis, B2 lesions involve the serosa, and B3 lesions extend to adjacent organs. C lesions designate lymph node involvement. C1 lesions involve mucosa or muscularis, whereas C2 lesions involve the serosa. Dukes' D lesions are metastatic. Approximate survival rates at 5 years for A lesions are 95%; for B1 lesions, 85%; for B2 lesions, 65%; for C1 lesions, 55%; and for C2 lesions, 25%. Stage D lesions have poor long-term survival rates.

HISTORY

Small neoplasms are often asymptomatic. Occult blood in the stool may be the only sign. As the size of the lesion grows, right colon lesions usually cause bleeding that is more significant, whereas lesions in the left colon typically present with obstructive symptoms, including a change in stool caliber, tenesmus, or constipation. Frank obstruction may also occur. Any lesion may produce crampy abdominal pain. Perforation

TABLE 4-1 TNM Staging Classification of Colorectal Cancer*

Stage	Description
TNM system	
Primary tumor (T)	
TX	Primary tumor cannot be assessed
T0	No evidence of tumor in resected specimen (prior polypectomy or fulguration)
Tis	Carcinoma in situ
T1	Invades into submucosa
T2	Invades into muscularis propria
T3/T4	Depends on whether serosa is present
Serosa present	
T3	Invades through muscularis propria into subserosa
	Invades serosa (but not through)
	Invades pericolic fat within the leaves of the mesentery
T4	Invades through serosa into free peritoneal cavity or through serosa into a contiguous organ
No serosa	(distal two thirds of rectum, posterior left or right colon)
T3	Invades through muscularis propria
T4	Invades other organs (vagina, prostate, ureter, kidney)
Regional lymph nodes (N)	
NX	Nodes cannot be assessed (e.g., local excision only)
N0	No regional node metastases
N1	1–3 positive nodes
N2	4 or more positive nodes
N3	Central nodes positive
Distant metastases (M)	
MX	Presence of distant metastases cannot be assessed
M0	No distant metastases
M1	Distant metastases present
Dukes' staging system correlated with TNM	
Dukes' A	T1, N0, M0
	T2, N0, M0
Dukes' B	T3, N0, M0
	T4, N0, M0
Dukes' C	T (any), N1, M0; T (any), N2, M0
Dukes' D	T (any), N (any), M1
MAC system correlated with TNM	
MAC A	T1, N0, M0
MAC B1	T2, N0, M0
MAC B2	T3, N0, M0; T4, N0, M0
MAC B3	T4, N0, M0
MAC C1	T2, N1, M0; T2, N2, M0
MAC C2	T3, N1, M0; T3, N2, M0
	T4, N1, M0; T4, N2, M0
MAC C3	T4, N1, M0; T4, N2, M0

TNM, tumor, nodes, metastases; MAC, modified Astler-Coller
*In all pathologic staging systems, particularly those applied to rectal cancer, the abbreviations *m* and *g* may be used; *m* denotes microscopic transmural penetration; *g* or *m + g* denotes transmural penetration visible on gross inspection and confirmed microscopically.

TNM definitions

Primary tumor (T)

TX	Primary tumor cannot be assessed
T0	No evidence of primary tumor
Tis	Carcinoma in situ: intraepithelial or invasion of the lamina propria*
T1	Tumor invades submucosa
T2	Tumor invades muscularis propria
T3	Tumor invades through the muscularis propria into the subserosa or into nonperitonealized pericolic or perirectal tissues
T4	Tumor directly invades other organs or structures and/or perforates visceral peritoneum**,***

* Tis includes cancer cells confined within the glandular basement membrane (intraepithelial) or lamina propria (intramucosal) with no extension through the muscularis mucosae into the submucosa.
** Direct invasion in T4 includes invasion of other segments of the colorectum by way of the serosa (e.g., invasion of the sigmoid colon by a carcinoma of the cecum).
*** Tumor that is adherent macroscopically to other organs or structures is classified T4. If no tumor is present in the adhesion microscopically, however, the classification should be pT3. The V and L substaging should be used to identify the presence or absence of vascular or lymphatic invasion.

(Continued)

■ TABLE 4-1 TNM Staging Classification of Colorectal Cancer* *(continued)*

Stage	Description
Regional lymph nodes (N)	
NX	Regional nodes cannot be assessed
N0	No regional lymph node metastasis
N1	Metastasis in 1–3 regional lymph nodes
N2	Metastasis in 4 or more regional lymph nodes

Note: A tumor nodule in the pericolorectal adipose tissue of a primary carcinoma without histologic evidence of residual lymph node in the nodule is classified in the pN category as a regional lymph node metastasis if the nodule has the form and smooth contour of a lymph node. If the nodule has an irregular contour, it should be classified in the T category and also coded as V1 (microscopic venous invasion) or V2 (if it was grossly evident), because there is a strong likelihood that is represents venous invasion.

Distant metastasis (M)	
MX	Distant metastasis cannot be assessed
M0	No distant metastasis
M1	Distant metastasis
AJCC stage groupings	
Stage 0	Tis, N0, M0
Stage I	T1, N0, M0
	T2, N0, M0
Stage IIA	T3, N0, M0
	Stage IIB
	T4, N0, M0
Stage IIIA	T1, N1, M0
	T2, N1, M0
Stage IIIB	T3, N1, M0
	T4, N1, M0
Stage IIIC	Any T, N2, M0
Stage IV	Any T, Any N, M1

Used with the permission of the American Joint Committee on Cancer (AJCC), Chicago, Illinois. The original source for this material is the AJCC Cancer Staging Manual, 6th ed. (2002), published by Springer-Verlag, New York, www.springeronline.com.

causes peritonitis. Constitutional symptoms, including weight loss, anorexia, and fatigue, are common.

PHYSICAL EXAMINATION

Rectal examination may reveal occult or gross blood. A mass may be palpable on abdominal examination.

Stigmata of hereditary disorders, including familial polyposis syndrome or Gardner's syndrome, may be present.

DIAGNOSTIC EVALUATION

Evaluation includes a hematocrit, which may show anemia. Carcinoembryonic antigen (CEA) should be drawn—though it is not a useful screening test, it is valuable as a marker for recurrent cancer. The liver is the most common site for metastases, and liver function tests can be abnormal in this case. Barium enema is an excellent test to demonstrate malignancy. Colonoscopy has the advantage of allowing biopsy or total excision of a lesion. CT is useful to evaluate for extent of disease and the presence of metastases (Fig. 4-2). Magnetic resonance imaging (MRI) may be better to evaluate liver metastases but usually does not add much to CT. Positron-emission tomography (PET) scan is useful for finding sites of metastases or recurrent disease in the setting of a rising CEA in a patient with a previous resection. For rectal lesions, endorectal ultrasound is the standard of care for assessing the depth of tumor invasion and the presence of lymph node metastases (Fig. 4-3).

TREATMENT

Therapy of colon cancer is based on surgical removal of the lesion. If the lesion can be removed endoscopically and pathologic evaluation reveals carcinoma in

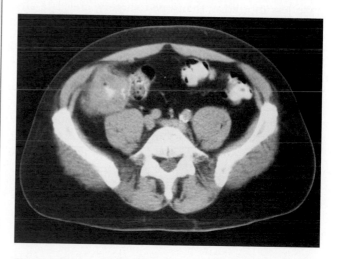

Figure 4-2 • Preoperative CT scan of a patient with cecal cancer invading the anterior abdominal wall and psoas muscle.
From Kelsen DP, Daly JM, Kern SE, Levin B, Tepper JE. *Gastrointestinal Oncology: Principles and Practice.* Philadelphia, PA: Lippincott Williams & Wilkins; 2002: 47–45.

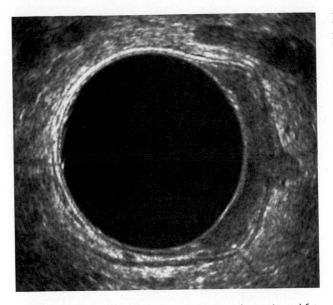

Figure 4-3 • uT3 lesion. There is invasion into the perirectal fat. The extension of the tumor into the perirectal fat is shown by a break in the outer white line and the thumbprinting of the tumor. From Kelsen DP, Daly JM, Kern SE, Levin B, Tepper JE. *Gastrointestinal Oncology: Principles and Practice.* Philadelphia, PA: Lippincott Williams & Wilkins; 2002: 46–45.

situ and complete excision, treatment is considered complete. For lesions that cannot be removed endoscopically, bowel resection is required. Segmental colon resection based on blood supply and lymphatic drainage is undertaken after suitable mechanical and antimicrobial cleansing. Laparoscopic approaches have less morbidity than open surgery, and data are accumulating that this approach is equally effective as open surgery in terms of long-term survival, though tumor recurrence continues to be of concern to some. The basic operation is the same regardless of the approach. Examples of the extent of resection for different types of colectomy are shown in Figure 4-4. For lesions that lie close to the anus, anastomosis may not be possible, and colostomy may be necessary. For stage C and probably stage B2 lesions, chemotherapy with 5-fluorouracil (5-FU) and levamisole is beneficial. Liver metastases should be resected if they number three or less and are easily accessible.

COLECTOMY: THE OPERATION

Preoperative preparation includes mechanical and antimicrobial bowel cleansing. Most resections are performed via a midline incision. The extent of excision for various tumors is described in Figure 4-4.

Mobilization of the right or left colon involves incising the white line of Toldt on the respective sides. Care is taken to avoid the ureter, which can be injured as the colon is mobilized. Consideration of a ureteral stent should be made if the tumor is bulky and there is concern about finding the ureter intraoperatively. The transverse colon is intraperitoneal and does not require mobilization. Once adequate length of colon has been mobilized, the peritoneum overlying the mesentery is incised to its root, and all the mesenteric vessels in the specimen are ligated. Noncrushing clamps are placed alongside the resection margin to reduce spillage, and the ends of the bowel are usually stapled and the specimen removed. Reconstruction of bowel continuity is performed with double-layer hand-sewn or single-layer stapled anastomosis. For low colon or rectal anastomosis, use of an EEA stapler placed through the anus is a preferred technique.

🔑 4-4 KEY POINTS

1. Colon cancer follows a progression from adenoma to carcinoma.
2. Adenomatous polyps are considered premalignant and must be removed entirely.
3. Screening for colon cancer involves a yearly stool test for occult blood and sigmoidoscopy every 3 to 5 years.

ANGIODYSPLASIA

Angiodysplasia is being recognized with increasing frequency as a significant source of lower gastrointestinal hemorrhage. These lesions most commonly occur in the cecum and right colon.

EPIDEMIOLOGY

Angiodysplasia is one of the most common causes of lower gastrointestinal bleeding. The prevalence increases with age to an incidence of approximately one fourth of the elderly.

HISTORY

Patients usually present with multiple episodes of low-grade bleeding. Ten percent of the time, patients present with massive bleeding.

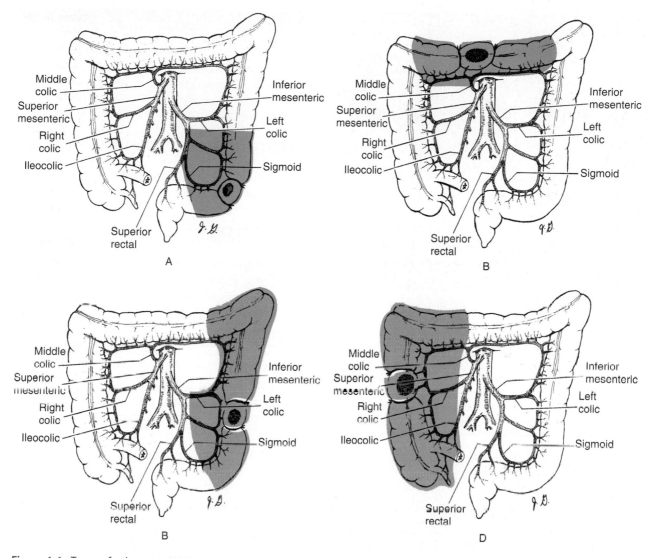

Figure 4-4 • Types of colectomy. (A) Sigmoid colectomy; **(B)** transverse colectomy; **(C)** left colectomy; **(D)** right colectomy.
Adapted from Kelsen DP, Daly JM, Kern SE, Levin B, Tepper JE. *Gastrointestinal Oncology: Principles and Practice*. Philadelphia, PA: Lippincott Williams & Wilkins; 2002: 47–4, 47–2, 47–3, 46–1.

DIAGNOSTIC EVALUATION

Diagnosis can be made with arteriography, nuclear scans, or colonoscopy.

TREATMENT

Endoscopy with laser ablation, electrocoagulation, or angiography with vasopressin is often effective. Because 80% of lesions rebleed, definitive treatment, which may require segmental colectomy, is recommended in most cases.

🔑 4-5 KEY POINT

1. Angiodysplasia is common in the elderly and is one of the most common causes of lower gastrointestinal bleeding.

VOLVULUS

A volvulus occurs when a portion of the colon rotates on the axis of its mesentery, compromising blood flow and creating a closed-loop obstruction (Fig. 4-5).

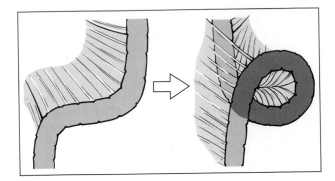

Figure 4-5 • Volvulus.

Because of their relative redundancy, the sigmoid (75%) and cecum (25%) are most commonly involved.

EPIDEMIOLOGY

The incidence of volvulus is approximately 2 in 100,000. Risk factors include age, chronic constipation, previous abdominal surgery, and neuropsychiatric disorders.

HISTORY

The patient usually relates the acute onset of crampy abdominal pain and distention.

PHYSICAL EXAMINATION

The abdomen is tender and distended, and peritoneal signs of rebound and involuntary guarding may be present. Frank peritonitis and shock may follow.

DIAGNOSTIC EVALUATION

Abdominal radiographs may reveal a massively distended colon and a "bird's beak" at the point of obstruction.

TREATMENT

Sigmoid volvulus may be reduced by rectal tube, enemas, or proctoscopy. Because of the high rate of recurrence, operative repair after the initial resolution is recommended. Treatment of cecal volvulus is usually operative at the outset, as nonoperative intervention is rarely successful.

🔑 4-6 KEY POINTS

1. Volvulus is a life-threatening condition that presents with abdominal pain and distention.
2. Abdominal radiographs may be diagnostic.

APPENDICITIS

Appendicitis is the most common reason for urgent abdominal operation.

EPIDEMIOLOGY

Young adults are most commonly affected. Appendicitis will develop in approximately 10% of people over their lifetime.

HISTORY

Patients typically complain of epigastric pain that migrates to the right lower quadrant. Anorexia is an almost universal complaint. The presence of generalized abdominal pain may signify rupture.

PHYSICAL EXAMINATION

Nearly all patients have right lower quadrant tenderness, classically located at McBurney's point, between the umbilicus and anterosuperior iliac spine. Rebound and guarding develop as the disease progresses and the peritoneum becomes inflamed. Low-grade fever is common. Rectal examination may reveal tenderness or a mass. Higher fever is associated with perforation. Signs of peritoneal irritation include the obturator sign (pain on external rotation of the flexed thigh) and the psoas sign (pain on right thigh extension).

DIAGNOSTIC EVALUATION

The white blood cell count is usually mildly elevated; high elevations are not usually seen unless perforation has occurred. Twenty-five percent of patients have abnormal urinalysis. Ultrasonographic evidence of appendicitis includes wall thickening, luminal distention, and lack of compressibility. Ultrasound is also useful for demonstrating ovarian pathology, which is in the differential diagnosis of women with right lower quadrant pain. Barium enema often shows non-filling of the appendix. CT may show inflammation in the area of the appendix.

TREATMENT

Uncomplicated appendicitis requires appendectomy. Both open and laparoscopic techniques are appropriate. Laparoscopic appendectomy is associated with shorter hospital course and faster return to work; however, costs are probably higher. Selected adults with appendiceal abscess who are clinically improving can be managed nonoperatively with antibiotics and CT-guided drainage. Children with perforated appendicitis require appendectomy with drainage of any abscess cavities.

🔑 4-7 KEY POINT

1. Appendicitis is the most common reason for urgent abdominal operation.

References

Chawla AK, Kachnic LA, Clark JW, Willett CG. Combined modality therapy for rectal and colon cancer. *Semin Oncol.* 2003;30(4 Suppl 9):101-112.

Davies MM, Larson DW. Laparoscopic surgery for colorectal cancer: the state of the art. *Surg Oncol.* 2004;13(2-3):111-118. Review.

Pituitary, Adrenal, and Multiple Endocrine Neoplasias

PITUITARY

ANATOMY AND PATHOPHYSIOLOGY

The pituitary gland is located at the base of the skull within the sella turcica, a hollow in the sphenoid bone. The optic chiasm lies anterior; the hypothalamus lies above; and cranial nerves III, IV, V, and VI and the carotid arteries lie in proximity. These structures are all at risk for compression or invasion from a pituitary tumor. Visual field defects can occur when a tumor encroaches on the optic chiasm. This most commonly presents as a bitemporal hemianopsia (Fig. 5-1). The gland weighs less than 1 g and is divided into an anterior lobe, or adenohypophysis (anterior adeno), and a posterior lobe, or neurohypophysis. The anterior pituitary produces its own hormones—prolactin, growth hormone (GH), follicle-stimulating hormone (FSH), luteinizing hormone (LH), adrenocorticotropin (ACTH), and thyrotropin—all under the control of hypothalamic hormones that travel directly from the hypothalamus through a portal circulation to the anterior pituitary (Fig. 5-2). The hormones of the posterior pituitary, vasopressin and oxytocin, are produced in the hypothalamus and are transported to the posterior lobe.

PROLACTINOMA

Pathology

Most prolactin-secreting tumors are not malignant. Prolactin-secreting tumors are divided into macroadenomas and microadenomas. Macroadenomas are characterized by gland enlargement, whereas microadenomas do not cause gland enlargement.

Epidemiology

Prolactinoma is the most common type of pituitary neoplasm. Macroadenomas are more common in men, whereas microadenomas are ten times more common in women.

History

Macroadenomas usually produce headache as the tumor enlarges. Women may describe irregular menses, amenorrhea, or galactorrhea.

Physical Examination

Defects of extraocular movements occur in 5% to 10% of patients and reflect compromise of cranial nerves III, IV, or VI. Women may have galactorrhea, whereas only 15% of men have sexual dysfunction or gynecomastia.

Diagnostic Evaluation

A serum prolactin level of greater than 300 µg/L establishes a diagnosis of pituitary adenoma, whereas a level above 100 µg/L is suggestive. Magnetic resonance imaging (MRI) differentiates microadenomas from macroadenomas and allows characterization of local tumor growth.

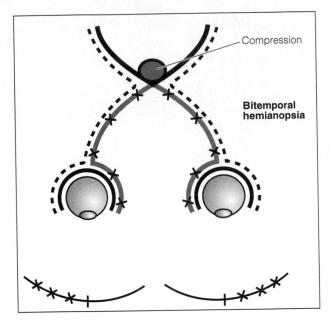

Figure 5-1 • Visual disturbances from compressive pituitary lesions.

Treatment

Asymptomatic patients with microadenomas can be followed without treatment. When symptoms of hyperprolactinemia occur, a trial of bromocriptine or cabergoline should be initiated. In the event of failure, transsphenoidal resection provides an 80% short-term cure rate, although long-term relapse may be as high as 40%. For patients who desire children, transsphenoidal resection provides a 40% success rate for childbearing.

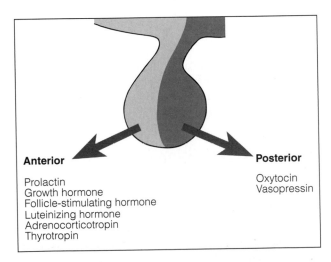

Figure 5-2 • Pituitary hormones.

Management options for macroadenomas with compressive symptoms include bromocriptine, which may decrease the size of the tumor, and surgical resection, often in combination. Resection is associated with high recurrence rates. Radiation therapy is effective for long-term control but is associated with panhypopituitarism.

🔑 5-1 KEY POINT

1. Prolactinoma is the most common pituitary tumor and is usually not malignant.

GROWTH HORMONE HYPERSECRETION

Pathogenesis

GH stimulates production of growth-promoting hormones, including somatomedins and insulinlike GH. Overproduction results in acromegaly, which is almost exclusively due to a pituitary adenoma, although abnormalities in hypothalamic production of GH-releasing hormone can also occur.

Epidemiology

Acromegaly has a prevalence of 40 per million.

History

Patients may complain of sweating, fatigue, headaches, voice changes, arthralgias, and jaw malocclusion. Symptoms usually develop over a period of years. The patient may have a history of kidney stones.

Physical Examination

The hallmark of the disease is bony overgrowth of the face and hands, with roughened facial features and increased size of the nose, lips, and tongue (Fig. 5-3). Signs of left ventricular hypertrophy occur in more than half of all patients, and hypertension is common.

Diagnostic Evaluation

Serum GH levels are elevated, and GH is not suppressed by insulin challenge. Insulin resistance may be present. An MRI should be obtained to delineate the extent of the lesion.

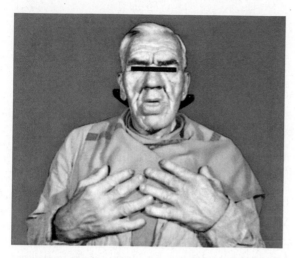

Figure 5-3 • Acromegaly is characterized by enlargement of the facial features (nose, ears) and the hands and feet.
From Weber J, Kelley J. *Health Assessment in Nursing*, 2nd ed. Philadelphia, PA: Lippincott Williams & Wilkins; 2003:D10.1a.

Treatment

Options include resection, radiation, and bromocriptine. Surgical cure rates are approximately 75% in patients with lower preoperative GH levels but only 35% in patients with high preoperative GH levels. Radiation is effective but slow and may result in panhypopituitarism. Bromocriptine can suppress GH production in combination with other treatment modalities; it is not usually effective as a single therapy.

5-2 KEY POINTS

1. The diagnosis of acromegaly is based on characteristic appearance and elevated growth hormone levels.
2. Treatment options include surgery, radiation, and bromocriptine.

FOLLICLE-STIMULATING HORMONE AND LUTEINIZING HORMONE HYPERSECRETION

Epidemiology

These tumors comprise approximately 4% of all pituitary adenomas.

History

Patients usually complain of headache or visual field changes from compression. Symptoms of panhypopituitarism may be present, as the tumors often grow to large size. Women have no symptoms that are attributable to oversecretion of FSH or LH. Men with FSH-secreting tumors may complain of depressed libido.

Physical Examination

The patient may have signs of compression.

Diagnostic Evaluation

Hormone levels are elevated.

Treatment

Surgery is necessary to relieve compression if it occurs.

THYROTROPIN AND ADRENOCORTICOTROPIN EXCESS

These diseases are discussed in their respective sections.

ADRENAL

ANATOMY AND PHYSIOLOGY

The adrenal glands lie just above the kidneys, anterior to the posterior portion of the diaphragm. The right gland is lateral and just posterior to the inferior vena cava, whereas the left gland is inferior to the stomach and near the tail of the pancreas. The blood supply derives from the superior supra-adrenal, the middle supra-adrenal, and the inferior supra-adrenal coming from the inferior phrenic artery, the aorta, and the renal artery respectively. Venous drainage on the right is to the inferior vena cava and on the left is to the renal vein.

The gland is divided into cortex and medulla. The cortex secretes glucocorticoids (cortisol), mineralocorticoids (aldosterone), and sex steroids, whereas the medulla secretes catecholamines (epinephrine, norepinephrine, and dopamine) (Fig. 5-4). Cholesterol is the precursor for both glucocorticoids and mineralocorticoids through a variety of pathways, beginning with the formation of pregnenolone, the rate-limiting step for corticoid synthesis.

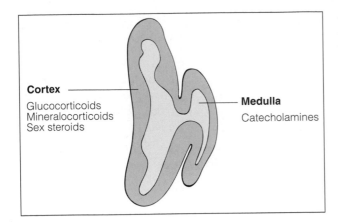

Figure 5-4 • Adrenal hormones.

Cortisol is secreted in response to ACTH from the pituitary, which is, in turn, controlled by corticotropin-releasing factor (CRF) secretion from the hypothalamus. Hypovolemia, hypoxia, hypothermia, and hypoglycemia stimulate cortisol production. Cortisol has many actions, including stimulation of glucagon release and inhibition of insulin release.

Exogenous glucocorticoids suppress the immune system and impair wound healing. They block inflammatory cell migration and inhibit antibody production, histamine release, collagen formation, and fibroblast function. These effects are significant causes of morbidity in patients maintained on steroid therapy.

Aldosterone secretion is controlled by the renin-angiotensin system. In response to decreased renal blood flow or hyponatremia, juxtaglomerular cells secrete renin. This causes cleavage of angiotensinogen to angiotensin I, which in turn is cleaved to angiotensin II. Angiotensin II causes vasoconstriction and stimulates aldosterone secretion. Aldosterone stimulates the distal tubule to reabsorb sodium. This increases water retention and works to restore circulating blood volume and pressure.

CUSHING SYNDROME

Pathogenesis

Cushing syndrome is due to overproduction of cortisol. In approximately 80% of patients, cortisol overproduction is secondary to ACTH hypersecretion. A pituitary adenoma is the cause in 80% of these patients (strictly termed *Cushing disease*), whereas the remainder derive from other tumors, including small-cell carcinoma of the lung and carcinoid tumors

of the bronchi and gut. Adrenal adenoma is the cause of cortisol hypersecretion in 10% to 20% of patients, whereas adrenal carcinoma and excess CRF production from the hypothalamus are unusual sources for increased cortisol production.

History

Patients may complain of weight gain, easy bruising, lethargy, and weakness.

Physical Examination

Patients have a typical appearance, with truncal obesity, striae, and hirsutism (Fig. 5-5). Hypertension, proximal muscle weakness, impotence or amenorrhea, osteoporosis, glucose intolerance, and ankle edema may be present.

Diagnostic Evaluation

Increased cortisol production is most reliably demonstrated by 24-hour urine collection. Low ACTH levels suggest an adrenal source, as the autonomously secreted cortisol suppresses ACTH production. The dexamethasone suppression test is useful in differentiating among pituitary microadenomas, macroadenomas, and ectopic sources of ACTH. Dexamethasone is a potent inhibitor of ACTH release. In patients with pituitary microadenomas, dexamethasone is able to suppress ACTH production, whereas in the

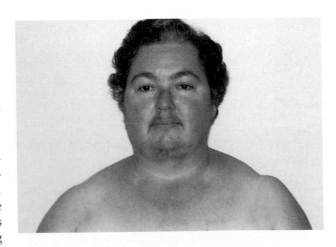

Figure 5-5 • Pheochromocytoma.

other patient groups, this effect is not seen. Response to corticotropin-releasing hormone (CRH) stimulation is accentuated when the source is pituitary but not when the source is adrenal or ectopic.

Treatment

Therapy is directed toward removing the source of increased cortisol production. For pituitary sources, resection is preferred. For an adrenal source, adrenalectomy is curative if the lesion is an adenoma. Resection should be attempted for adrenal carcinoma.

🔑 5-3 KEY POINT

1. Cushing syndrome results from overproduction of cortisol, most commonly due to adrenocorticotropin overproduction from a pituitary tumor.

HYPERALDOSTERONISM

Pathogenesis

Causes of excess secretion of aldosterone include adrenal adenoma (80%), idiopathic bilateral hyperplasia (15%), adrenal carcinoma (rare), or ectopic production (rare).

Epidemiology

The prevalence among patients with diastolic hypertension is 1 in 200.

History

Symptoms are usually mild and include fatigue and nocturia.

Physical Examination

Hypertension is the most common finding.

Diagnostic Evaluation

Hypokalemia occurs as sodium is preferentially reabsorbed in the distal tubule, causing kaliuresis. Aldosterone levels in serum and urine are increased, and serum renin levels are decreased. If hyperaldosteronism is demonstrated, computed tomography (CT) or MRI is used to evaluate the adrenals. In this setting, the presence of a unilateral adrenal mass greater than 1 cm strongly suggests the diagnosis of adrenal neoplasm.

Treatment

Surgical excision is indicated for adenoma, whereas excision or debulking, or both, and chemotherapy are the treatment of choice for carcinoma. Pharmacologic therapy for patients with idiopathic bilateral hyperplasia usually includes a trial of potassium-sparing diuretics and dexamethasone.

🔑 5-4 KEY POINT

1. Adrenal adenoma is the most common cause of hyperaldosteronism.

EXCESS SEX STEROID PRODUCTION

Adrenal neoplasms can secrete excess sex steroids. Virilization suggests the lesion is malignant. Treatment is surgical removal.

ADRENAL INSUFFICIENCY

Pathogenesis

Long-term steroid use can lead to suppression of the adrenal cortex. In the setting of surgical stress, the cortex may not be able to respond with the appropriate release of glucocorticoids and mineralocorticoids. These patients are at risk for Addison disease or acute adrenal insufficiency, which is life-threatening.

History

Patients complain of abdominal pain and vomiting.

Physical Examination

Obtundation may occur. Hypotension, hypovolemia, and hyperkalemia can lead to shock and cardiac arrhythmias.

Treatment

Preoperative identification of patients at risk for adrenal suppression is critical, and perioperative steroids are necessary. The steroids should be continued if the patient is in critical condition.

PHEOCHROMOCYTOMA

Pathophysiology

This tumor produces an excess of catecholamines.

Epidemiology

Pheochromocytoma is a rare tumor. It occurs most commonly in the third and fourth decades, with a slight female predominance. Approximately 5% to 10% occur in association with syndromes, including the multiple endocrine neoplasias types IIa and IIb. Approximately 10% are malignant. Pheochromocytoma is the etiology of hypertension in fewer than 0.2% of patients. The catecholamine source is most commonly the adrenals but can occur elsewhere in the abdomen (10%) or outside the abdomen (2%).

History

Patients may complain of headaches, tachycardia or palpitations, anxiety, sweating, chest or abdominal pain, and nausea either in paroxysms or constant in nature. Physical exertion, tyramine-containing foods, nicotine, succinylcholine, and propranolol can precipitate attacks.

Diagnostic Evaluation

Systolic blood pressure can be marked by peaks approaching 300 mm Hg but may be normal on a single reading. Diagnosis is established by elevated urinary epinephrine and norepinephrine, as well as their metabolites, metanephrine, normetanephrine, and vanillylmandelic acid. CT or MRI yields information about tumor size and location. (Fig. 5-6) Nuclear medicine scan using radioactive metaiodobenzylguanidine is especially useful for finding extra-adrenal tumors.

Treatment

Pheochromocytomas are removed surgically. Preoperative preparation is critical to ensure that the patient does not have a hypertensive crisis in the operating room.

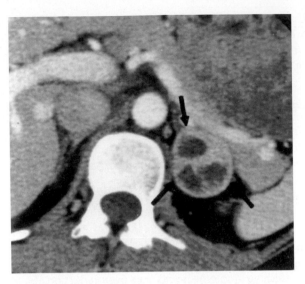

Figure 5-6 • Cushing syndrome.

Alpha blockade with phenoxybenzamine or phentolamine is usually combined with beta blockade. It is important to establish alpha blockade first. Isolated beta blockade in the setting of catecholamine surge can produce shock, as cardiac function is prevented from increasing while systemic vascular resistance increases.

INCIDENTAL ADRENAL MASS

Approximately 1% of CT scans obtained for any reason reveal an adrenal mass, making the incidental adrenal mass a common clinical scenario. Workup includes a thorough history to find symptoms of Cushing syndrome, hyperaldosteronism, or pheochromocytoma. Laboratory evaluation includes urine for 24-hour urinary-free cortisol; dexamethasone suppression test; serum sodium and potassium; and epinephrine, norepinephrine, and their metabolites. Resection is recommended for evidence of metabolite activity either by symptoms or by laboratory evaluation or if the mass is larger than 4 cm.

5-7 KEY POINT

1. Incidental adrenal masses should be excised if they have symptomatic or biochemical evidence of activity or if they are greater than 4 cm in diameter.

MULTIPLE ENDOCRINE NEOPLASIAS

Multiple endocrine neoplasia (MEN) I consists of the three p's: parathyroid hyperplasia, pancreatic islet cell tumors, and anterior pituitary adenomas. Parathyroid hyperplasia occurs in 90% of cases. Pancreatic neoplasms occur in 50%. These are most commonly gastrinoma, but tumors of cells producing insulin, glucagon, somatostatin, and vasoactive intestinal peptide can also occur. The anterior pituitary tumor is most commonly prolactin-secreting and occurs in approximately 25% of patients. MEN IIa consists of medullary thyroid carcinoma (MTC), pheochromocytoma, and parathyroid hyperplasia. MTC occurs in almost all affected patients. MEN IIb consists of MTC, pheochromocytoma, and mucosal neuromas, with characteristic body habitus, including thick lips, kyphosis, and pectus excavatum. Diagnosis and treatment follow treatment for the individual lesions (Table 5-1).

TABLE 5-1 Multiple Endocrine Neoplasias (MEN)

MEN I
Parathyroid hyperplasia
Pancreatic islet cell tumors
Anterior pituitary adenoma
MEN IIa
MTC
Pheochromocytoma
Parathyroid hyperplasia
MEN IIb
MTC
Pheochromocytoma
Mucosal neuromas

MTC, medullary thyroid carcinoma.

5-8 KEY POINTS

1. Multiple endocrine neoplasia (MEN) I consists of parathyroid hyperplasia, pancreatic islet cell tumors, and anterior pituitary adenomas.
2. MEN IIa consists of medullary thyroid carcinoma (MTC), pheochromocytoma, and parathyroid hyperplasia.
3. MEN IIb consists of MTC, pheochromocytoma, and mucosal neuromas.

References

Chanson P, Salenave S. Diagnosis and treatment of pituitary adenomas. *Minerva Endocrinol.* 2004;29(4): 241–275.

Lenders JW, Eisenhofer G, Mannelli M, Pacak K. Phaeochromocytoma. *Lancet.* 2005;366(9486):665–675.

Shapiro SE, Cote GC, Lee JE, Gagel RF, Evans DB. The role of genetics in the surgical management of familial endocrinopathy syndromes. *J Am Coll Surg.* 2003;197(5):818–831.

Esophagus

ANATOMY AND PHYSIOLOGY

The esophagus extends from the pharynx to the stomach, bounded posteriorly by the vertebral column and thoracic duct, anteriorly by the trachea, laterally by the pleura, and on the left by the aorta. It courses downward to the left, then to the right, and back to the left to join the stomach. The vagus nerve forms a plexus around the esophagus, which condenses to form two trunks on the lateral esophagus. These trunks, in turn, rotate so that the left trunk moves anteriorly while the right trunk moves posteriorly.

The esophageal mucosa is lined by squamous epithelium that becomes columnar near the gastroesophageal junction. The next layer encountered moving radially outward is the submucosa, which contains the Meissner plexus. Next are two muscular layers separated by the Auerbach plexus. There is no true serosa, unlike in the stomach, small intestine, and colon.

The superior and inferior thyroid arteries supply the upper esophagus, whereas the intercostals, left gastric, and phrenic arteries supply the lower esophagus. Venous drainage of the upper esophagus is into the inferior thyroid and vertebrals; the mid and lower esophagus drains into the azygous, hemiazygous, and left gastric veins. Submucosal veins can become engorged in patients with portal hypertension, causing varices and potentially life-threatening bleeding. Lymphatics drain into cervical, mediastinal, celiac, and gastric nodes. Innervation is from the vagus, cervical sympathetic ganglion, splanchnic ganglion, and celiac ganglion. These are responsible for esophageal motility.

Peristasis conveys food into the stomach. Gastric reflux is prevented by increased tone in the lower portion of the esophagus; there is no true sphincter. Air ingestion is prevented by resting tone in the upper esophagus.

ESOPHAGEAL NEOPLASMS

Pathology

Esophageal neoplasms are almost always malignant. Benign tumors account for fewer than 1% of cases. Benign lesions include leiomyomas, hemangiomas, cysts, or polyps. Worldwide, most esophageal cancers are of squamous cell histology, but the incidence of adenocarcinoma predominates in the United States.

Pathogenesis

Mucosal insult seems to be a common pathway toward the genesis of esophageal cancer. As such, chronic ingestion of extremely hot liquids, esophageal burns from acid or base ingestions, radiation-induced esophagitis, and reflux esophagitis are all implicated in causing esophageal cancer. Alcohol, cigarettes, nitrosamines, and malnutrition also play a role in the development of cancer. Barrett esophagus, which occurs when the normal squamous epithelium becomes columnar in response to injury, is considered a premalignant lesion. Patients with Plummer-Vinson syndrome also have a higher incidence of esophageal cancer.

Epidemiology

The incidence of esophageal cancer varies according to the presence of the etiologic factors described previously. For example, in places with high soil nitrosamine content, the prevalence of esophageal cancer is almost 1% of adults. In the United States, the incidence of esophageal cancer is 4 in 100,000 white males and 12 in 100,000 black males. It is most commonly a disease of men between 50 and 70 years of age.

History

The classic presentation of esophageal adenocarcinoma is progressive dysphagia to solids in an older male with a history of gastroesophageal reflux disease (GERD). Typically, patients feel well and have no other symptoms. Occasionally patients may have mild weight loss, more often related to diminished caloric intake due to obstructive symptoms than to cachexia from metastatic disease. Chest pain and odynophagia are relatively infrequent.

Patients with esophageal squamous cell carcinoma often have a history of heavy alcohol and tobacco use and present with more pronounced symptoms due to more advanced disease.

Physical Examination

Signs are nonspecific, and patients appear well unless significant metastatic disease is present. Supraclavicular lymphadenopathy at presentation is rare.

Diagnostic Evaluation

Barium esophagogram detects malignant lesions in 96% of patients. This is usually the initial study for the evaluation of new onset dysphagia. Definitive diagnosis requires tissue confirmation by flexible esophagoscopy with biopsy. To determine the stage of the primary tumor and regional nodal status, some centers utilize endoscopic esophageal ultrasound (EUS). Evaluation of regional or distant disease is done by combined chest/abdominal computed tomography (CT) scan and occasionally fluorodeoxyglucose positron emission tomography (FDG-PET) scan.

Staging

The TNM (tumor-node-metastasis) system is used for staging esophageal cancer. Clinical stage (cTNM) is determined by evaluation of all information derived from physical examination, imaging studies, endoscopy, biopsy, and occasionally laparoscopy or thoracoscopy. Once the clinical stage is determined, rational treatment plans can be proposed to the patient (Table 6-1 and Fig. 6-1).

Treatment

Because there is no serosa, disease is often locally invasive or metastatic on presentation, leading to poor overall survival statistics. Current treatment employs

■ TABLE 6-1 AJCC TNM Classification of the Esophagus

Primary Tumor (T)

TX	Primary tumor cannot be assessed
T0	No evidence of primary tumor
Tis	Carcinoma in situ
T1	Tumor invades lamina propria or submucosa
T2	Tumor invades muscularis propria
T3	Tumor invades adventitia
T4	Tumor invades adjacent structures

Regional Lymph Nodes (N)

NX	Regional lymph nodes cannot be assessed
T0	No regional lymph node metastasis
T1	Regional lymph node metastasis

Distant Metastasis (M)

MX	Distant metastasis cannot be assessed
M0	No distant metastasis
M1	Distant metastasis
	Tumors of the lower thoracic esophagus:
M1a	Metastasis in celiac lymph nodes
M1b	Other distant metastasis
	Tumors of the midthoracic esophagus:
M1a	Not applicable
M1b	Nonregional lymph nodes and/or other distant metastasis
	Tumors of the upper thoracic esophagus:
M1a	Metastasis in cervical nodes
M1b	Other distant metastasis

Stage Grouping

Stage 0	Tis	N0	M0
Stage I	T1	N0	M0
Stage IIA	T2	N0	M0
	T3	N0	M0
Stage IIB	T1	N1	M0
	T2	N1	M0
Stage III	T3	N1	M0
	T4	Any N	M0
Stage IV	Any T	Any N	M1
Stage IVA	Any T	Any N	M1a
Stage IVB	Any T	Any N	M1b

(Continued)

TABLE 6-1 AJCC TNM Classification of the Esophagus *(continued)*	
Histologic Grade (G)	
Gx	Grade cannot be assessed
G1	Well differentiated
G2	Moderately differentiated
G3	Poorly differentiated
G4	Undifferentiated

Used with permission of the American Joint Committee on Cancer (AJCC), Chicago, Illinois. Original source: AJCC Cancer Staging Manual, 6th ed. New York, NY: Springer-Verlag; 2002.

🔑 6-1 KEY POINTS

1. The esophagus lacks a true serosa, and therefore cancer is often not contained at the time of diagnosis. Overall survival remains poor.
2. Most esophageal tumors are malignant.
3. Risk factors for esophageal cancer include Barrett esophagus from gastroesophageal reflux disease, burns, and nitrosamines.
4. Current therapy is multimodal.

radiation, chemotherapy, and surgery. For contained local disease, esophagectomy provides the possibility of cure. Some evidence has shown that induction chemotherapy and radiotherapy preoperatively, followed by surgery, can improve long-term survival, but this remains an area of controversy.

ACHALASIA

Pathophysiology

Achalasia results from absence of peristalsis and failure of the lower esophageal sphincter to relax with swallowing. The cause of this seems to reside in the Auerbach plexus, but the exact mechanism is not well understood.

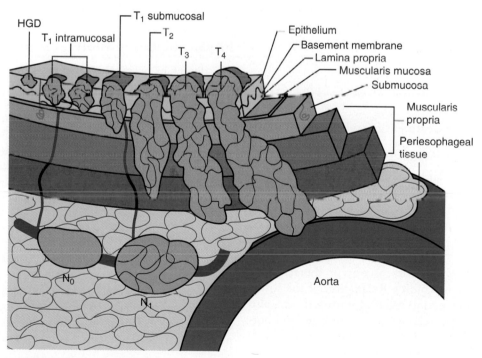

No regional lymph node metastases = N_0
Regional lymph node metastases present = N_1
High grade dysplasia = HGD

Figure 6-1 • Visual representation of TNM staging of esophageal cancer.
Reprinted with permission of The Cleveland Clinic Foundation.

Epidemiology

Achalasia is the most common esophageal motility disorder, with an incidence of 6 per 100,000. Men and women are equally affected. Patients usually present in the fourth through sixth decades.

History

Patients complain of dysphagia. As ingested material is unable to pass into the stomach, a column of food or liquid rises in the esophagus. When there is a change to a recumbent position, liquid spills into the mouth or into the lungs, and patients may complain of regurgitation or have a history of pneumonia. Because the regurgitant does not include gastric contents, it is not sour tasting.

Diagnostic Evaluation

Esophagography demonstrates distal narrowing. Dynamic video imaging reveals abnormal peristalsis. The lower portion of the esophagus may taper to form a "bird's beak" appearance, and there may be proximal dilation. Motility and pressure studies confirm the diagnosis. Esophagoscopy should also be performed to rule out cancer and to evaluate for strictures.

Treatment

The most effective treatment for relieving symptoms of dysphagia caused by achalasia is surgical. Esophagomyotomy (Heller myotomy) is usually performed using the laparoscopic approach with low morbidity. Longitudinal separation of the esophageal musculature is carried from the distal esophagus onto the proximal stomach, and partial fundoplication is often performed to reduce postoperative gastroesophageal reflux. Myotomy can also be performed through the chest by thoracoscopy or thoracotomy, but with greater morbidity. Relaxation of the lower esophageal sphincter and relief of symptoms can also be achieved by repeated endoscopic injections of botulinum toxin (Botox). Results are inferior and short-lasting. Pneumatic balloon dilatation of the lower esophageal sphincter is another option but also has inferior results and carries the risk of esophageal perforation. Surgical therapy provides superior long-term results over medical interventions.

🔧 6-2 KEY POINTS

1. Achalasia is the most common disorder of esophageal motility.
2. It can usually be differentiated from cancer by esophagoscopy, but complete evaluation for malignancy should be undertaken.

PERFORATION

Etiology

Esophageal perforation occurs most commonly after instrumentation (iatrogenic) but also from ingested foreign bodies or penetrating trauma. Spontaneous esophageal rupture occurring after an episode of vomiting is known as Boerhaave syndrome.

History

Recent instrumentation of the upper airway or esophagus should raise the possibility of esophageal injury. Boerhaave syndrome should be suspected in cases involving recent emesis. Epigastric abdominal pain and shoulder pain are frequent complaints.

Physical Examination

The degree of presenting symptoms is usually proportional to the time from when perforation occurred. Subcutaneous emphysema is often found, as well as, abdominal tenderness or distention. If a major delay in diagnosis has occurred (i.e., due to lack of history in an unconscious patient), then fever, tachycardia, and hypotension due to sepsis is common. The presence of a hydropneumothorax can result in diminished breath sounds over the involved hemithorax.

Diagnostic Evaluation

Chest x-ray can demonstrate pleural effusion, hydropneumothorax, and mediastinal emphysema. An esophageal contrast study can confirm the location of perforation. If diagnosis is still uncertain, then intraluminal examination by flexible endoscopy can also be utilized. Thoracentesis can reveal empyema.

Treatment

Immediate exploratory thoracotomy and repair of the perforation is indicated in almost all cases. Pleural space drainage with chest tubes continues postoperatively. Small cervical lacerations can be managed with antibiotics alone and close observation. Mortality due to esophageal perforation is more than 50% if any injury to the thoracic esophagus is not treated within 24 hours.

6-3 KEY POINT

1. Esophageal perforation is frequently fatal if not diagnosed and treated early.

References

Enzinger PC, Mayer PJ. Esophageal cancer. *N Engl J Med*. 2003;349:2241–2252.

Pearson, et al. *Esophageal Cancer*. Philadelphia, PA: Churchill Livingstone; 2002:655–945.

Thomas, CR. Current and ongoing progress in the therapy for resectable esophageal cancer. *Dis Esophagus*;18(4):211–214.

Gallbladder

ANATOMY AND PHYSIOLOGY

The gallbladder is located in the right upper quadrant of the abdomen beneath the liver. The cystic duct exits at the neck of the gallbladder and joins the common hepatic duct to form the common bile duct, which empties into the duodenum at the ampulla of Vater (Fig. 7-1). This is surrounded by the sphincter of Oddi, which regulates bile flow into the duodenum. Bile produced in the liver is stored in the gallbladder. Cholecystokinin stimulates gallbladder contraction and release of bile into the duodenum. The spiral valves of Heister prevent bile reflux into the gallbladder. Arterial supply is from the cystic artery, which most commonly arises from the right hepatic artery and courses through the triangle of Calot, which is bounded by the cystic duct, the common hepatic duct, and the edge of the liver.

GALLSTONE DISEASE

Cholelithiasis is the presence of gallstones. Biliary colic is pain produced when the gallbladder contracts against a stone in the neck of the gallbladder or as a stone passes through the bile ducts. Acute cholecystitis refers to inflammation and infection of the gallbladder; total or partial occlusion of the cystic duct is thought to be required. The most common organisms cultured during an episode of acute cholecystitis are *Escherichia coli*, *Klebsiella*, enterococci, *Bacteroides fragilis*, and *Pseudomonas*. Choledocholithiasis refers to stones in the common bile duct (Fig. 7-2).

PATHOGENESIS

Stones can be composed of cholesterol, calcium bilirubinate, or both. Cholesterol stones make up approximately 80% of stones in Western countries.

Stone formation occurs when bile becomes supersaturated with cholesterol. Stones then precipitate out of solution. A high-cholesterol diet causes increased concentrations of cholesterol and probably has a role in the pathogenesis of cholesterol stones. Calcium bilirubinate (pigment stones) are found in association with chronic biliary infection, cirrhosis, and hemolytic processes, such as sickle cell anemia, thalassemia, and spherocytosis.

EPIDEMIOLOGY

Approximately 10% of the U.S. population has gallstones. They are more common in women; other risk factors include obesity, multiparity, diabetes, and age over the fifth decade. Spinal cord injury predisposes to cholesterol stones. Gallstones are a major cause of pancreatitis.

HISTORY

Most patients with gallstones are asymptomatic. Patients with biliary colic usually complain of right upper quadrant or epigastric pain, often radiating around the right side or to the back. The pain is usually postprandial, occurring after eating. Pain episodes may be precipitated by fatty food intake and last several hours before resolving. Concurrent nausea and vomiting are common.

Cholecystitis implies infection and inflammation. The pain of cholecystitis is usually constant, with progressive worsening. Patients may have fever, chills, or sweats.

Choledocholithiasis can result in transient or complete blockage of the common bile duct. Patients may relate episodes of passing dark urine or light-colored stools caused by the inability of bile pigments to reach the gastrointestinal tract and from subsequent renal clearance. Choledocholithiasis can also lead to ascending cholangitis, demonstrated by right upper quadrant abdominal pain, fever, and chills.

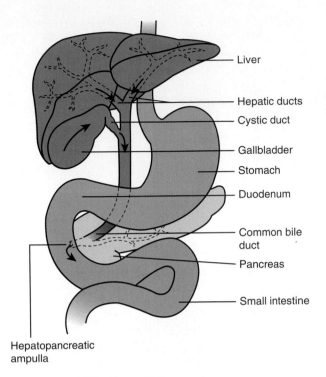

Liver

Hepatic ducts

Cystic duct

Gallbladder

Stomach

Duodenum

Common bile duct

Pancreas

Small intestine

Hepatopancreatic ampulla

Figure 7-1 • Gallbladder and biliary anatomy.

Pancreatitis due to choledocholithiasis (gallstone pancreatitis) typically manifests with epigastric pain radiating to the back.

PHYSICAL EXAMINATION

Physical examination in simple biliary colic reveals right upper quadrant tenderness but usually no fever. Cholecystitis may be associated with fever and signs of peritoneal irritation, including right upper quadrant rebound and guarding. The classic finding in acute cholecystitis is the arrest of inspiration on deep right upper quadrant palpation as pressure from the examiner's hand contacts the inflamed gallbladder and peritoneum (the Murphy sign). Choledocholithiasis may be associated with jaundice, in addition to signs of biliary colic. Cholangitis is classically marked by fever, right upper quadrant pain, and jaundice (the Charcot triad). Progression of cholangitis to sepsis defines Reynolds pentad by adding hypotension and mental status changes. Patients in whom gallstone pancreatitis has developed exhibit epigastric tenderness.

DIAGNOSTIC EVALUATION

Laboratory examination in biliary colic is often unremarkable. Cholecystitis usually manifests with increased white blood cell count. Choledocholithiasis is associated with increased serum bilirubin and alkaline phosphatase. Cholangitis usually causes elevated serum bilirubin and transaminase levels. Gallstone pancreatitis is accompanied by elevations in serum amylase and lipase.

Ultrasound has a sensitivity and specificity of 98% for gallstones. The stones present as an opacity, with an echoless shadow posteriorly (Fig. 7-3). Moving the patient demonstrates migration of the stones to the dependent portion of the gallbladder. Ultrasound can also be used to detect acute cholecystitis. Fluid around the gallbladder, a thickened gallbladder wall, and gallbladder distention all support the diagnosis of acute cholecystitis.

When ultrasound is equivocal or acalculous cholecystitis is suspected, cholescintigraphy (e.g., HIDA [hepatobiliary iminodiacetic acid] scan) is almost 100% sensitive and 95% specific for acute cholecystitis. In this test, a radionucleotide that is injected intravenously is taken up in the liver and excreted into the biliary tree. If the cystic duct is obstructed, as in acute cholecystitis, the gallbladder does not fill, and the radionucleotide passes directly into the duodenum.

Common duct stones are best identified by endoscopic retrograde cholangiopancreatography (ERCP), which is performed using an endoscope to visualize the

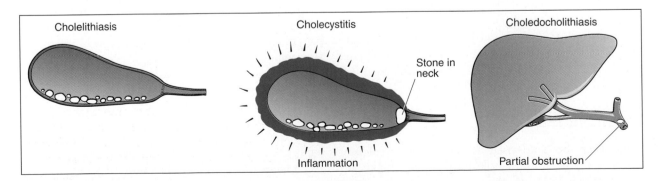

Cholelithiasis

Cholecystitis

Stone in neck

Inflammation

Choledocholithiasis

Partial obstruction

Figure 7-2 • Biliary pathology.

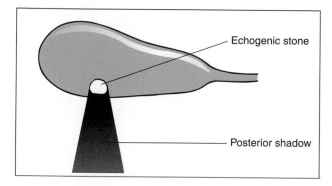

Figure 7-3 • Gallbladder ultrasound—cholelithiasis.

ampulla where the pancreatic and biliary ducts enter the duodenum. Contrast is passed retrograde and outlines the biliary tree and pancreatic ducts (Fig. 7-4). Magnetic resonance cholangiopancreatography (MRCP) is an emerging technology that can noninvasively detect common bile duct stones; however, it lacks the therapeutic capabilities of ERCP for stone extraction.

COMPLICATIONS

Gallstone pancreatitis may occur due to a common duct stone causing blockage of the ampulla, theoretically resulting in bile reflux into the pancreatic duct

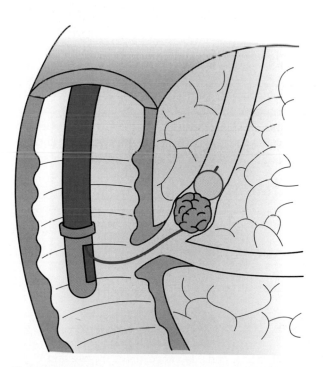

Figure 7-4 • ERCP removal of common bile duct stone using balloon-tip catheter.

or increased intraductal pressure. Delay in diagnosis of cholecystitis often results in gallbladder necrosis. Emphysematous cholecystitis due to *Clostridium perfringens* can be seen in diabetic patients. A large gallstone may erode the gallbladder wall and cause a fistula to form between the gallbladder and bowel (duodenum or colon). The large stone can then pass through the fistula into the bowel, resulting in distal bowel obstruction (gallstone ileus).

TREATMENT

For patients with asymptomatic stones found on workup for other problems, the incidence of symptoms or complications is approximately 2% per year. Cholecystectomy is usually not advised for these patients. For individuals with biliary colic, laparoscopic cholecystectomy is a safe and effective procedure. This is ideally done in an elective setting, after the patient's symptoms resolve. If the preoperative workup suggests that common duct stones may be present, either ERCP or intraoperative cholangiography should be considered.

Patients with acute cholecystitis should be resuscitated with fluids, because vomiting and infection are likely to have caused dehydration. Broad-spectrum intravenous antibiotics should be administered. Laparoscopic cholecystectomy is the procedure of choice in the acute setting, although it tends to be more difficult and has a higher rate of conversion to open technique compared with the elective situation. For patients who are too ill to tolerate cholecystectomy, a cholecystostomy tube should be considered. This involves placing a percutaneous drain into the gallbladder for decompression and drainage. Cholecystectomy can then be performed when the patient is stable.

Patients with gallstone pancreatitis require fluid resuscitation and observation. Mild episodes account for 80% of cases. Intravenous antibiotics are only indicated in severe cases with pancreatic necrosis, infected necrosis, or infectious complications. Early ERCP is indicated in patients with signs of common bile duct obstruction (cholangitis, jaundice, dilated common duct on imaging studies) and in patients with severe disease. Once pancreatic inflammation subsides, cholecystectomy with intraoperative cholangiography should be performed during the same hospitalization to reduce the risk of recurrent pancreatitis and to rule out residual common duct stones. If stones are present, intraoperative common duct exploration or postoperative ERCP are done. The risk of recurrent pancreatitis is approximately 40% within 6 weeks.

Cholangitis due to choledocholithiasis requires rapid diagnosis and treatment. Intravenous antibiotics and urgent biliary decompression and drainage are indicated. ERCP with sphincterotomy is the primary intervention. Other methods of decompression include percutaneous drainage by interventional radiology or open surgical drainage.

🔑 7-1 KEY POINTS

1. Cholelithiasis refers to stones in the gallbladder; symptoms typically include right upper quadrant pain.
2. Cholecystitis implies inflammation and infection in the gallbladder; symptoms typically include right upper quadrant pain and signs of infection.
3. Choledocholithiasis refers to stones in the common bile duct, and patients often have increased bilirubin.
4. Cholangitis refers to infection in the small ducts of the liver, and patients often have right upper quadrant pain, fever, and jaundice.
5. Pancreatitis is a serious complication of gallstone disease.

CANCER OF THE GALLBLADDER

EPIDEMIOLOGY

Cancer of the gallbladder is three times more common in females. The incidence is 2.5 in 100,000. Risk factors include gallstones, porcelain gallbladder, and adenoma. Large gallstones carry greater risk.

PATHOLOGY

Approximately 80% are adenocarcinomas, 10% are anaplastic, and 5% are squamous cell.

HISTORY

Patients usually present with vague right upper quadrant pain. Weight loss and anorexia may also be present.

PHYSICAL EXAMINATION

A right upper quadrant mass may be present. Jaundice represents invasion or compression of the biliary system.

TREATMENT

Options include radical resection of the gallbladder, including partial hepatic resection, or palliative operation as symptoms arise.

PROGNOSIS

Unless the cancer is found incidentally at cholecystectomy for stones, only 4% of patients will be alive in 5 years.

BILE DUCT CANCERS

EPIDEMIOLOGY

Bile duct cancers are rare. Risk factors include ulcerative colitis, sclerosing cholangitis, and infection with *Clonorchis sinensis*.

HISTORY

Patients with advanced disease typically complain of right upper quadrant pain.

PHYSICAL EXAMINATION

The patient may have a distended gallbladder or jaundice, as the tumor obstructs the biliary tree.

DIAGNOSTIC EVALUATION

Ultrasound and computed tomography show evidence of obstruction, but percutaneous transhepatic cholangiography (PTC) or ERCP is usually necessary to demonstrate the lesion. Patients with sclerosing cholangitis should be followed closely for evidence of cancer.

TREATMENT

Treatment consists of surgical resection.

PROGNOSIS

Mortality is 90% at 5 years.

🔑 7-2 KEY POINT

1. Gallbladder and bile duct cancers are rare and usually fatal.

References

Ahmed A, Cheung RC, Keefe EB. Management of gallstones and their complications. *Am Fam Physician*. March 2000;61(6):1673–1680, 1687–1688.

Kalloo AN, Kantsevoy, SV. Gallstones and biliary disease. *Primary Care*. September 2001;28(3):vii, 591–606.

Moscati, RM. Cholelithiasis, cholecystitis, and pancreatitis. *Emerg Med Clin North Am*. November 1996;14(4):719–737.

ANATOMY

Coronary circulation begins at the sinus of Valsalva where the right and left coronary arteries (RCA, LCA) arise. The left main (LM) artery branches into the left anterior descending (LAD) and the left circumflex (LCX) arteries. The LAD supplies the anterior of the left ventricle, the apex of the heart, the intraventricular septum, and the portion of the right ventricle that borders the intraventricular septum. The LCX travels in the groove separating the left atrium and ventricle and gives off marginal branches to the left ventricle. The RCA travels between the right atrium and ventricle to supply the lateral portion of the right ventricle (Fig. 8-1). The posterior descending artery (PDA) comes from the RCA in 90% of patients and supplies the arteriovenous node. Patients whose PDA arises from the RCA are termed right dominant. If the PDA arises from the left circumflex, the system is left dominant.

The aortic valve is located between the left ventricle and the aorta. It usually has three leaflets, which form three sinuses. One sinus gives rise to the RCA, another to the LCA, and the third forms the noncoronary sinus. The mitral valve is located between the left atrium and ventricle. It normally has two leaflets, with the anterior protruding farther across the valve. Chordae tendineae attach the leaflets to the papillary muscles, which in turn serve to tether the leaflets to the ventricular wall.

CORONARY ARTERY DISEASE

EPIDEMIOLOGY

Atherosclerosis of the coronary arteries is the most common cause of mortality in the United States, responsible for one third of all deaths. Approximately five million Americans have coronary artery disease (CAD), which is five times more prevalent in males than in females. Risk factors include hypertension, family history, hypercholesterolemia, smoking, obesity, diabetes, and physical inactivity.

PATHOPHYSIOLOGY

Coronary artery stenosis is a gradual process that begins in the second decade. When the lumen decreases to 75% of the native area, the lesion becomes hemodynamically significant.

HISTORY

Patients with ischemic heart disease usually complain of substernal chest pain or pressure that may radiate down the arms or into the jaw, teeth, or back. Typically, the pain occurs during periods of physical exertion or emotional stress. Episodes that are reproducible and resolve with rest are termed *stable angina*. If the pain occurs at rest or does not improve with rest, is new and severe, or is progressive, it is termed *unstable angina* and suggests impending infarction.

PHYSICAL EXAMINATION

The patient may have evidence of peripheral vascular disease, including diminished pulses. Signs of ventricular failure, including cardiomegaly, congestive heart failure, an S3 or S4, or murmur of mitral regurgitation (MR), may occur.

DIAGNOSTIC EVALUATION

The electrocardiogram (ECG) may show signs of ischemia or an old infarct. A chest radiograph may

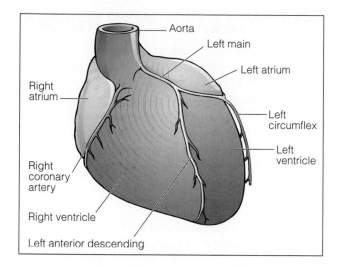

Figure 8-1 • Coronary anatomy.

show an enlarged heart or pulmonary congestion. An exercise stress test is sensitive in identifying myocardium at risk. These areas can be localized using nuclear medicine scans, including thallium imaging. Echocardiography is extremely useful in evaluating myocardial function and valvular competence. Angiography is the gold standard for identifying lesions in the coronary arteries, assessing their severity, and planning operative intervention.

TREATMENT

Patients with severe disease of the LM or with severe disease in the three major coronary arteries have decreased mortality after coronary artery bypass surgery. Pain is reliably relieved in more than 85% of patients. Surgical options include bypass using the internal mammary arteries or saphenous veins. Internal mammary bypass is preferred because of higher patency rates.

🔑 8-1 KEY POINTS

1. Coronary artery disease (CAD) is the leading cause of mortality in the United States.
2. Risk factors include hypertension, smoking, obesity, diabetes, hypercholesterolemia, inactivity, and family history.
3. CAD is treated surgically if all three coronary arteries or the left main coronary artery are diseased or if patients have debilitating symptoms.

AORTIC STENOSIS

ETIOLOGY

Aortic stenosis (AS) can present early in life—for example, when the valve is unicuspid—but more commonly occurs in the older population. A congenitally bicuspid valve usually causes AS by the time the patient reaches 70 years of age. Other causes include rheumatic fever, which results in commissural fusion and subsequent calcification, and degenerative stenosis, in which calcification occurs in the native valve.

PATHOPHYSIOLOGY

The initial physiologic response to AS is left ventricular hypertrophy to preserve stroke volume and cardiac output. Left ventricular hypertrophy and increasing resistance at the level of the valve result in decreased cardiac output, pulmonary hypertension, and myocardial ischemia.

HISTORY

Patients often complain of angina, syncope, and dyspnea, with dyspnea being the worst prognostic indicator.

PHYSICAL EXAMINATION

A midsystolic ejection murmur, as well as cardiomegaly and other signs of congestive heart failure, may be present. Pulsus tardus et parvus, a delayed, diminished impulse at the carotid, may be apparent.

DIAGNOSTIC EVALUATION

Echocardiography or cardiac catheterization reliably studies the valve. A decrease in the aortic valve area from the normal 3 or 4 cm to less than 1 cm signifies severe disease.

TREATMENT

Patients who are symptomatic should undergo aortic valve replacement unless other medical conditions make it unlikely that the patient could survive the operation. In asymptomatic individuals, progressive cardiomegaly is an indication for operation, as surgical therapy is superior to medical therapy.

8-2 KEY POINTS

1. Aortic stenosis can be caused by a congenital bicuspid valve or rheumatic fever.
2. Symptoms include angina, syncope, and dyspnea.

8-3 KEY POINTS

1. Aortic insufficiency can be caused by rheumatic fever, endocarditis, connective tissue disorders, aortic dissection, and trauma.
2. Symptoms include angina and dyspnea.

AORTIC INSUFFICIENCY

ETIOLOGY

Aortic insufficiency (AI) can be caused by rheumatic fever, connective tissue disorders including Marfan and Ehlers-Danlos syndromes, endocarditis, aortic dissection, and trauma.

PATHOPHYSIOLOGY

The incompetent valve causes a decrease in cardiac output, and left ventricular dilatation occurs. The larger ventricle is subject to higher wall stress, which increases myocardial oxygen demand.

HISTORY

Patients complain of angina or symptoms of systolic dysfunction.

PHYSICAL EXAMINATION

Typically, there is a crescendo-decrescendo diastolic murmur and a wide pulse pressure with a water hammer quality. The point of maximal impulse (PMI) may be displaced or diffuse.

DIAGNOSTIC EVALUATION

Echocardiography is a sensitive and specific means of making the diagnosis.

TREATMENT

Symptomatic patients should undergo replacement surgery if their medical condition allows them to tolerate a major procedure.

MITRAL STENOSIS

ETIOLOGY

Mitral stenosis (MS) develops in 40% of patients with rheumatic heart disease. Rheumatic heart disease occurs after pharyngitis caused by group A streptococcus. A likely autoimmune phenomenon causes pancarditis, resulting in fibrosis of valve leaflets. Histologic findings include Aschoff nodules. MS may also be due to malignant carcinoid and systemic lupus erythematosus.

PATHOPHYSIOLOGY

Fibrosis progresses over a period of two or three decades, causing fusion of the leaflets, which take on a characteristic "fish mouth" appearance, significantly impeding blood flow through the valve. Increased left atrial pressures lead to left atrial hypertrophy, which in turn may cause atrial fibrillation or pulmonary hypertension. Pulmonary hypertension can further progress to right ventricular hypertrophy and right-sided heart failure.

EPIDEMIOLOGY

MS has a female predominance of 2:1.

HISTORY

Characteristic complaints include dyspnea and fatigability. Occasionally, pulmonary hypertension leads to hemoptysis.

PHYSICAL EXAMINATION

Cachexia or symptoms of congestive heart failure may be present with pulmonary rales and tachypnea. Jugular venous distention, peripheral edema, ascites, and a sternal heave of right ventricular hypertrophy may be appreciable. Heart sounds are usually characteristic, consisting of an opening snap followed by a low rumbling murmur. The splitting of the second heart sound is decreased, and the pulmonary component is louder. The heart rate may demonstrate the irregular pattern of atrial fibrillation.

DIAGNOSTIC EVALUATION

Chest x-ray may show cardiomegaly, including signs of left atrial hypertrophy. Pulmonary edema may be present. ECG may show atrial fibrillation. Broad, notched P waves are an indication of left atrial hypertrophy. Right axis deviation is evidence of right ventricular hypertrophy. Echocardiography with Doppler flow measurement is extremely useful for demonstrating MS, estimating flow, and assessing the presence of thrombi. Cardiac catheterization gives a direct measurement of transvalvular pressure gradient, from which the area of the mitral annulus can be calculated.

THERAPY

Surgical options include valvulotomy or replacement. Therapy is indicated for symptomatic patients.

🔑 8-4 KEY POINTS

1. Mitral stenosis is most commonly caused by rheumatic fever.
2. Symptoms include fatigue and dyspnea.

MITRAL REGURGITATION

ETIOLOGY

Approximately 40% of cases are due to rheumatic fever; other causes include idiopathic calcification associated with hypertension, diabetes, AS, and renal failure. Mitral valve prolapse progresses to MR in 5% of affected individuals. Less common causes include myocardial ischemia, trauma, endocarditis, and hypertrophic cardiomyopathy.

PATHOPHYSIOLOGY

As regurgitation becomes hemodynamically significant, the left ventricle dilates to preserve cardiac output. A significant volume is ejected retrograde, increasing cardiac work, left atrial volumes, and pulmonary venous pressure. This, in turn, may lead to left atrial enlargement and fibrillation or cause pulmonary hypertension, which could result in right ventricular failure.

EPIDEMIOLOGY

MR is more common than MS and has a male predominance.

HISTORY

Patients commonly complain of dyspnea, orthopnea, and fatigue.

PHYSICAL EXAMINATION

Patients may appear cachectic. Frequently, there is an irregular pulse, pulmonary rales, and a sternal heave. The pulse characteristically has a rapid upstroke, and waves may be present. A holosystolic murmur that radiates to the axilla or back is common. The PMI is often displaced.

DIAGNOSTIC EVALUATION

Chest x-ray may show cardiomegaly and pulmonary edema. ECG commonly demonstrates left ventricular or biventricular hypertrophy, left atrial enlargement, and P mitrale. Echocardiography is extremely useful in establishing the diagnosis and the underlying lesion. Cardiac catheterization is useful in establishing pulmonary pressures and cardiac output.

TREATMENT

Medical therapy consists of afterload reducing agents, such as angiotensin-converting enzyme (ACE) inhibitors, nitroglycerin, and diuretics. Surgical intervention is indicated if congestive failure interferes with daily life, if pulmonary hypertension or left ventricular dilation worsens, or if atrial fibrillation develops. If life-threatening MR develops from endocarditis, ischemia, or trauma, aggressive treatment with afterload reduction; a balloon pump, if necessary; and antibiotics, if indicated; should be used to convert an emergency operation to an elective one. Because of the severe hemodynamic instability that can occur, operative intervention involving repair or replacement may be necessary in the acute setting. These emergency operations carry greater than 15% mortality.

8-5 KEY POINTS

1. Mitral regurgitation is caused by rheumatic fever, idiopathic calcification, mitral valve prolapse, myocardial ischemia, trauma, endocarditis, and hypertrophic cardiomyopathy.
2. Symptoms include fatigue and dyspnea.

References

Bojar RM. *Manual of Perioperative Care in Adult Cardiac Surgery*. 4th ed. Oxford, UK: Blackwell Publishers; 2004.

Edmunds LH, Cohn LH, eds. *Cardiac Surgery in the Adult*. 2nd ed. New York, NY: McGraw-Hill Professional; 2003.

Hernias

A hernia occurs when a defect or weakness in a muscular or fascial layer allows tissue to exit a space in which it is normally contained. Hernias are categorized as reducible, incarcerated, or strangulated. Reducible hernias can be returned to their body cavity of origin. Incarcerated hernias cannot be returned to their body cavity of origin. Strangulated hernias contain tissue with a compromised vascular supply. These are particularly dangerous because they lead to tissue necrosis. If the bowel is involved, this can progress to perforation, sepsis, and death.

EPIDEMIOLOGY

Between 500,000 and 1,000,000 hernia repairs are performed each year. Five percent of people have an inguinal hernia repair during their lifetime. Half of all hernias are indirect inguinal, and one fourth are direct inguinal. In decreasing incidence are incisional and ventral (10%), femoral (6%), and umbilical (3%). Obturator hernias are rare. Indirect inguinal hernias are the most common in both males and females; overall, hernias have a 5:1 male predominance. Femoral hernias are more common in females than in males.

INGUINAL HERNIAS

ANATOMY

The abdominal contents are kept intraperitoneal by three fascial layers: The innermost layer is the transversalis, the middle layer is the internal oblique, and the outer layer is the external oblique. The transversalis and internal oblique, with the pubic tubercle, border the internal ring. The superior aspect of the ring is formed by the arch of the transversalis.

During normal development, the testes begin in an intraperitoneal position and descend through the internal ring, taking with them a layer of peritoneum that is stretched into a hollow tube called the *processus vaginalis*. This path taken by the testes could also be taken by the bowel—two things occur to prevent this. First, the processus vaginalis collapses from a tube into a cord. Next, the transversalis maintains the integrity of the ring. An indirect inguinal hernia occurs when the processus vaginalis fails to obliterate. In this case, bowel or other abdominal contents can escape from their intraperitoneal location. A direct hernia occurs when the transversalis becomes weakened, allowing abdominal contents to herniate directly through the fascia (Fig. 9-1). The external oblique, which inserts onto the pubic tubercle and bounds the external ring, has no function in the pathogenesis of hernias.

HISTORY

Patients with reducible inguinal hernias describe an intermittent bulge in the groin or scrotum. Persistence of the bulge with nausea or vomiting raises concern for incarceration. Severe pain at the hernia site or in the abdomen, with nausea or vomiting, may occur with strangulation.

PHYSICAL EXAMINATION

A finger is placed at the pubic tubercle and pushed upward to find the superficial ring; a bulge or pressure as the patient coughs or bears down may be felt. Reducible hernias can be pushed back into the abdomen; incarcerated hernias cannot. Strangulated hernias are tender, possibly with abdominal distention or signs of peritoneal irritation, including rebound pain and guarding.

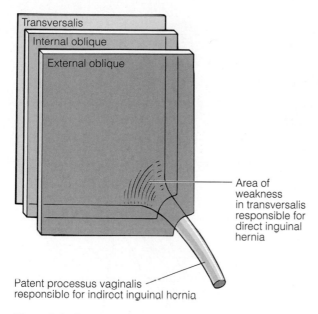

Transversalis

Internal oblique

External oblique

Area of weakness in transversalis responsible for direct inguinal hernia

Patent processus vaginalis responsible for indirect inguinal hernia

Figure 9-1 • Anatomy of inguinal hernias.

TREATMENT

The indications for hernia repair are to prevent bowel obstruction due to incarceration of intestine, prevent bowel strangulation and perforation, and relieve symptoms of hernia discomfort. Modern hernioplasty is based on the idea of a tensionfree repair utilizing an implantable biocompatible prosthesis, usually polypropylene.

Reducible inguinal hernias can be repaired on an elective basis. Both open and laparoscopic techniques are used. The usual indications for laparoscopic repair are bilaterality and recurrence. When a hernia is not reducible with gentle pressure, a trial of Trendelenburg position, sedation, and more forceful pressure can be attempted. If the hernia is thought to be strangulated, then reduction is contraindicated, because reducing necrotic bowel into the abdomen may produce bowel perforation and subsequent lethal sepsis. Emergency surgery is indicated in this situation.

UMBILICAL HERNIAS

Umbilical hernias occur at the umbilicus and are congenital. Most resolve spontaneously by the age of 2.

EPIDEMIOLOGY

The incidence is 10% of Caucasians and 40% to 90% of African Americans.

HISTORY

The patient may have a bulge at the umbilicus.

TREATMENT

Indications for operation include incarceration, strangulation, or cosmetic concerns. Because large hernias may become incarcerated, they should be repaired.

OTHER HERNIAS

Femoral hernias occur through the femoral canal (Fig. 9-2). Incisional hernias occur through a surgical incision, often as a result of infection. Ventral hernias occur in the midline. Internal hernias, a major cause of bowel obstruction, occur in patients after abdominal operations, when bowel gets trapped as a result of adhesions or new anatomic relationships. Obturator hernias, typically found in thin, elderly women, occur through the obturator canal, which admits the obturator nerve, artery, and vein. Most are asymptomatic, but nerve compression can result in paresthesias or pain radiating down the medial thigh (the Howship-Romberg sign).

These hernias are often incarcerated on presentation, usually causing small bowel obstruction. Treatments for all of the above hernias are based on the principles outlined.

🔑 9-1 KEY POINTS

1. Hernias are extremely common; inguinal hernias are the most common, and 5% of people require repair during their lifetime.
2. Indirect inguinal hernias, based on the internal ring, are more common than direct hernias.
3. Hernias that become incarcerated should be operated on urgently.
4. Hernias that become strangulated are a surgical emergency.
5. Umbilical hernias are congenital, more common in African Americans, and frequently resolve spontaneously.
6. Other hernia types include femoral, ventral, incisional, and internal.

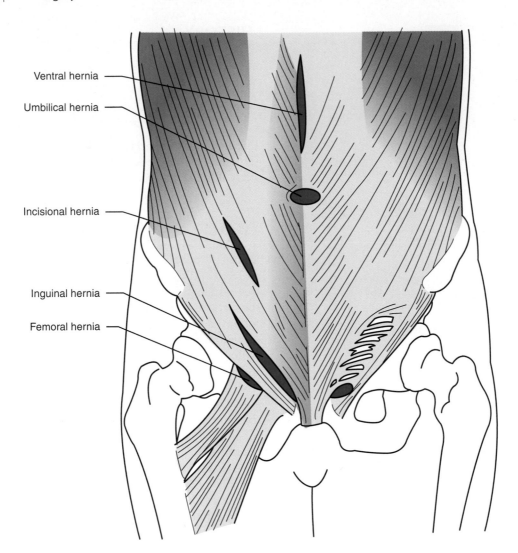

Figure 9-2 • Types of hernias.

References

Awad SS, Fagan SP. Current approaches to inguinal hernia repair. *Am J Surg.* 2004;188 (suppl 6A):3S-8S.

Avusse C, Delattre JF, Flament JB. The inguinal rings. *Surg Clin North Am.* 2000;80(1):49–69.

Fitzgibbons RJ Jr, Giobbie-Hurder A, Gibbs JO, et al. Watchful waiting vs. Repair of Inguinal Hernia in minimally symptomatic men: A Randomized clinical trial. *JAMA* 2006;295:285–292.

Flum, D.R. The Asymptomatic Hernia. *JAMA* 2006;295:328–329.

Macintyre IMC. Inguinal hernia repair. *Jr Coll Surg Edinburgh.* 2001;46(6):349–353.

ANATOMY

The kidneys are retroperitoneal structures. They are surrounded by Gerota's fascia and lie lateral to the psoas muscles and inferior to the posterior diaphragm. Blood supply is by renal arteries; usually, there is a single renal artery, but there may be more than one. The renal veins drain into the inferior vena cava. The ureters course retroperitoneally, dorsal to the cecum on the right and the sigmoid colon on the left. They cross the iliac vessels at the bifurcation between internal and external and enter the true pelvis to empty into the bladder. The bladder lies below the peritoneum in the true pelvis and is covered by a fold of peritoneum. Blood supply is from the iliac arteries through the superior, middle, and inferior vesical arteries. Sympathetic nerve supply is from L1 and L2 roots, whereas parasympathetic is from S2, S3, and S4.

STONE DISEASE

ETIOLOGY

The most common kidney stones are calcium phosphate and calcium oxalate (80%); struvite (15%), uric acid (5%), and cystine (1%) are other causes. Calcium stones are usually idiopathic but can be caused by hyperuricosuria and hyperparathyroidism. Struvite stones are caused by infection with urease-producing organisms, usually *Proteus*. Uric acid stones are common in patients with gout and can occur with Lesch-Nyhan syndrome or tumors. Cystine stones are hereditary.

EPIDEMIOLOGY

Approximately 20% of males and 10% of females will be affected by nephrolithiasis over their lifetime.

Calcium stones and struvite stones are more common in women, uric acid stones are twice as common in men, and cystine stones occur with equal frequency in men and women.

HISTORY

Stone formation is associated with a number of dietary factors, which should be investigated. Low fluid intake is a general risk factor. Diets high in salt promote excretion and increased urinary concentration of calcium. High intake of animal protein results in increased calcium, uric acid, citrate, and acid excretion. Low-calcium diets can also be problematic, as they increase oxalate excretion.

Patients with stone disease usually present with acute onset of pain beginning in the flank and radiating down to the groin, although the pain can be anywhere along this track. The patient is often unable to find a comfortable position, and vomiting is common. Dysuria, frequency, and hematuria may be described.

DIAGNOSTIC EVALUATION

Workup includes evaluation of urinary sediment that shows hematuria, unless the affected ureter is totally obstructed. Crystals are frequently observed. It is imperative to determine the type of stone to guide therapy. Urinary sediment may be extremely useful for this purpose. Calcium oxalate stones are either dumbbell-shaped or bipyramidal and may be birefringent. Uric acid crystals are small and red-orange. Cystine stones are flat, hexagonal, and yellow. Struvite stones are rectangular prisms. Uric acid crystals and calcium oxalate crystals can be found in normal individuals and thus are less useful when found in the sediment.

Blood work should evaluate for elevated serum calcium and uric acid. Measurement of parathyroid hormone levels should be performed in patients with hypercalcemia or high urinary calcium.

An abdominal radiograph should be obtained, as calcium, struvite, and cystine stones are all radiopaque. Intravenous pyelography involves intravenous administration of an iodinated dye that is excreted in the kidneys. This allows diagnosis of stones by outlining defects in the ureter or demonstrating complete obstruction due to stone disease. Retrograde pyelography involves injecting dye through the urethra and is useful for assessing the degree and level of obstruction. Ultrasonography of the kidneys can demonstrate the stone (Fig. 10-1) and hydronephrosis indicative of ureteral obstruction. The presence of fluid jets at the entrance of the ureter in the bladder precludes the diagnosis of total obstruction.

TREATMENT

In the acute setting, pain and nausea should be controlled with narcotics and antiemetics. Most stones pass spontaneously; deflazacort and nifedipine or tamsulosin may be used to facilitate stone passage. Stone size predicts spontaneous passage: Asymptomatic stones less than 5 mm usually do not require intervention.

Stones greater than 5 mm should be considered for intervention. Less invasive options include extracorporeal shock wave lithotripsy (ESWL); percutaneous nephrolithotomy (PCNL); and endoscopic lithotripsy using ultrasonic, electrohydraulic, or laser energy to remove stones. ESWL is the most common approach and involves using high-energy shock waves that originate extracorporeally. Focusing the energy on the stone causes fragmentation, which facilitates passage. This technique is not ideal for struvite or staghorn calculi. PCNL involves placement of a nephrostomy tube and is more efficacious than ESWL for stones that are large, complex, or composed of cysteine. PCNL and ESWL can be combined (Fig. 10-2). Open pyelolithotomy is reserved for patients who fail multiple attempts at less invasive approaches.

To prevent recurrent stones, patients should be counseled to increase fluid intake. Dietary modifications should be recommended based on the stone type. Pharmacologic interventions include a thiazide diuretic for patients with hypercalciuria and allopurinol or potassium citrate for uric acid stones. Hypocitraturia may be treated with potassium citrate. Oxalate stones may be treated with calcium if urinary calcium is low.

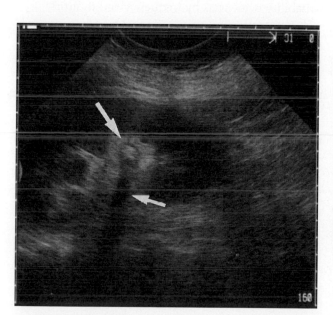

Figure 10-1 • Posterior shadowing: a stone within the renal pelvis (large arrow) casts a posterior shadow (small arrow).
From Harwood-Nuss A, Wolfson AB, et al. *The Clinical Practice of Emergency Medicine.* 3rd ed. Philadelphia, PA: Lippincott Williams & Wilkins; 2001:128.1.

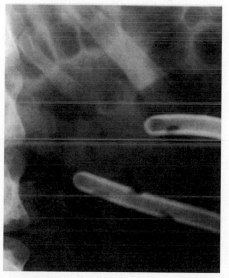

Figure 10-2 • Combined PCNL and ESWL for staghorn calculi. This 35-year-old woman presented with a *Proteus* urinary tract infection and was found to have a large complete left staghorn calculus. A second PCNL was then performed, requiring a second nephrostomy tube to effect complete stone removal.
From Harwood-Nuss A, Wolfson AB, et al. *The Clinical Practice of Emergency Medicine.* 3rd ed. Philadelphia, PA: Lippincott Williams & Wilkins; 2001:63-65.

1. Kidney stones are usually composed of calcium salts.
2. Symptoms include severe flank pain, which may radiate to the groin.
3. Stones greater than 5 mm should be considered for intervention. Most patients will respond to minimally invasive methods of stone removal.

RENAL CANCER

EPIDEMIOLOGY

Two percent of cancer deaths are attributable to renal cancer. Males are affected twice as often as females, and smoking may be a risk factor.

PATHOLOGY

Tumors are categorized as granular cell, tubular adenocarcinoma, Wilms tumor, or sarcoma.

HISTORY

Patients may experience hematuria and flank pain, which can be sudden in the event of hemorrhage. Fever and extrarenal pain from metastatic disease may be present. Approximately 30% of patients will present with metastatic disease.

PHYSICAL EXAMINATION

Tumors may be palpable.

DIAGNOSTIC EVALUATION

Intravenous pyelography demonstrates a defect in the renal silhouette. Computed tomography can differentiate between cystic and solid lesions.

TREATMENT

Initial treatment in most cases is radical nephrectomy with attempt to remove all tumor. For patients with metastatic disease, results with chemotherapy are disappointing. Gemcitabine and fluorouracil demonstrate limited activity against the tumor. Interleukin-2 is a drug approved by the Food and Drug Administration for renal cell cancer. Response rates are in the 15% to 20% range.

1. Renal cancer is responsible for 2% of cancer deaths, and treatment in most cases is radical nephrectomy.

BLADDER CANCER

PATHOLOGY

Transitional cell tumors make up 90% of bladder malignancies. The remainder are squamous cell and adenocarcinoma.

EPIDEMIOLOGY

Men are more frequently affected than women, by a ratio of 3:1. Smoking, beta-naphthylamine, and paraminophenol all predispose a person to the development of bladder cancer.

HISTORY

Most patients present with hematuria. Urinary tract infections (UTIs) are relatively common, as is bladder irritability evidenced by frequency and dysuria.

DIAGNOSTIC EVALUATION

Urinary cytology may reveal the presence of bladder cancer. Cystoscopy with biopsy confirms the diagnosis. Excretory urography may demonstrate the lesion.

TREATMENT

For local disease, transurethral resection with chemotherapy, including doxorubicin, mitomycin C, or thiotepa, is effective. For locally advanced disease, radical cystectomy (including prostatectomy in men) is combined with radiation and gemcitabine and cisplatin.

1. Patients with bladder cancer usually have hematuria.
2. Treatment may be transurethral resection for local disease; radical cystectomy is used for advanced disease.

References

Atala A. What's new in urology. *J Am Coll Surg.* 2004;199(3):446–461.

Curti BD. Renal cell carcinoma. *JAMA.* 2004;292(1):97–100.

Liver

ANATOMY AND PHYSIOLOGY

The liver is located in the right upper quadrant of the abdomen, bounded superiorly and posteriorly by the diaphragm; laterally by the ribs; and inferiorly by the gallbladder, stomach, duodenum, colon, kidney, and right adrenal. It is covered by Glisson's capsule and peritoneum. The right and left lobes of the liver are defined by the plane formed by the gallbladder fossa and the inferior vena cava. The falciform ligament between the liver and diaphragm is a landmark between the lateral and medial segments of the left lobe. The coronary ligaments continue laterally from the falciform and end at the right and left triangular ligaments. These ligaments define the bare area of the liver, an area devoid of peritoneum. The liver parenchyma is divided into eight segments based on arterial and venous anatomy (Fig. 11-1).

The hepatic circulation is based on a portal circulation that provides the liver with first access to all intestinal venous flow. Seventy-five percent of total hepatic blood flow is derived from the portal vein, which is formed from the confluence of the splenic and superior mesenteric veins. The remaining blood supply comes from the hepatic artery via the celiac axis. The right hepatic artery arises from the superior mesenteric artery in 15% of patients, and the left hepatic arises from the left gastric in 15% of patients. Blood leaving the liver enters the inferior vena cava via the right, middle, and left hepatic veins.

The liver is the site of many critical events in energy metabolism and protein synthesis. Glucose is taken up and stored as glycogen, and glycogen is broken down, as necessary, to maintain a relatively constant level of serum glucose. The liver is able to initiate gluconeogenesis during stress, and the liver can oxidize fatty acids to ketones, which the brain can use as an energy source. Proteins synthesized in the liver include the coagulation factors fibrinogen, prothrombin, prekallikrein, high-molecular-weight kininogen, and factors V, VII, VIII, IX, X, XI, and XII. Of these, prothrombin and factors VII, IX, and X are dependent on vitamin K. The anticoagulant warfarin (Coumadin) affects these vitamin K–dependent pathways, resulting in an increased prothrombin time. Albumin and alpha globulin are produced solely in the liver.

The liver's digestive functions include bile synthesis and cholesterol metabolism. Heme is used to form bilirubin, which is excreted in the bile after conjugation with glycine or taurine. Bile emulsifies fats to aid their digestion and plays a role in vitamin uptake. Bile salts excreted into the intestine are reabsorbed into the portal circulation. This cycle of bile excretion and absorption is termed the *enterohepatic circulation*. Total body bile circulates approximately ten times per day in this loop. Greater than 95% of excreted bile is reabsorbed, and the remainder must be resynthesized. The rate-limiting step of cholesterol synthesis involving the enzyme HMG–CoA (3-hydroxy-3-methyl-glutaryl–coenzyme A) reductase occurs in the liver, as does cholesterol metabolism to bile salts.

Detoxification occurs in the liver through two pathways: Phase I reactions involve cytochrome P450 and include oxidation, reduction, and hydrolysis. Phase II reactions consist of conjugation. These reactions are critical to destruction or renal clearance of toxins. The dosing of all oral drugs is determined only after considering the first-pass effect of the drug through the liver. The initial hydroxylation of vitamin D occurs in the liver. Immunologic functions are mediated by Kupffer cells, the resident liver macrophages.

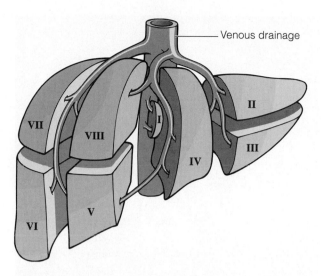

Venous drainage

I
II
III
IV
V
VI
VII
VIII

Figure 11-1 • Segmental anatomy of the liver.

BENIGN LIVER TUMORS

PATHOLOGY

Benign liver tumors include hepatocellular adenoma, focal nodular hyperplasia, hemangioma, and lipoma. Hemangiomas are categorized into capillary and cavernous types, the former being of no clinical consequence and the latter capable of attaining large size and rupturing.

EPIDEMIOLOGY

Only 5% of liver tumors are benign, with hemangioma the most common. Approximately 7% of people have a cavernous hemangioma at autopsy. The incidence of adenoma is one per million. Oral contraceptive use multiplies this risk by 40. Adenoma and focal nodular hyperplasia are five times more common in females.

HISTORY

Patients with adenomas and hemangiomas can be asymptomatic or present with dull pain; rupture can produce sudden onset of severe abdominal pain. These lesions can also become large enough to cause jaundice or symptoms of gastric outlet obstruction, including nausea and vomiting. Focal nodular hyperplasia is rarely symptomatic.

PHYSICAL EXAMINATION

Large lesions can be palpated. Jaundice may occur in patients if the tumor causes bile duct obstruction.

DIAGNOSTIC EVALUATION

These lesions are most often found incidentally at laparotomy or on imaging studies requested for other reasons. Laboratory evaluation is often unremarkable, although hemorrhage in an adenoma can lead to hepatocellular necrosis and a subsequent rise in transaminase levels. Hemangioma can cause a consumptive coagulopathy. Ultrasound differentiates cystic from solid lesions. Triple-phase computed tomography (CT) is the best study to distinguish between various types of benign and malignant lesions, but in certain cases, this determination is not possible. Adenomas are typically low-density lesions; focal nodular hyperplasias may appear with a filling defect or central scar, whereas hemangiomas have early peripheral enhancement after contrast administration. Hemangiomas should not be biopsied because of the risk of bleeding.

TREATMENT

Patients with adenoma who are using oral contraceptives should stop. If the lesion does not regress, resection should be considered in otherwise healthy individuals because of the risk of malignant degeneration or hemorrhage. Relative contraindications to resection include a tumor that is technically difficult to resect or tumors of large size in which a large portion of the liver would need to be removed. Symptomatic hemangiomas should be resected, if possible. Because focal nodular hyperplasia is not malignant and rarely causes symptoms, it should not be resected unless it is found incidentally at laparotomy and is small and peripheral enough to be wedged out easily.

LIVER CANCER

PATHOLOGY

Liver cancers are hepatomas, also known as hepatocellular carcinoma, or metastases from other primaries.

EPIDEMIOLOGY

Ninety-five percent of liver tumors are malignant. Hepatoma is one of the most common malignancies in the world, but rates in the United States are relatively low (approximately 2 per 100,000). It is more common in males than in females.

ETIOLOGY

Cirrhosis is a predisposing factor to hepatoma; as such, hepatitis B, the leading cause of cirrhosis, and alcoholism are associated with hepatoma development. Fungal-derived aflatoxins have been implicated as causes of hepatoma, as have hemochromatosis, smoking, vinyl chloride, and oral contraceptives.

HISTORY

Patients with hepatoma may complain of weight loss, right upper quadrant or shoulder pain, and weakness. Hepatic metastases are often indistinguishable from primary hepatocellular carcinoma.

PHYSICAL EXAMINATION

Hepatomegaly may be appreciable, and signs of portal hypertension, including splenomegaly and ascites, may be present. Jaundice occurs in approximately half of patients.

DIAGNOSTIC EVALUATION

Laboratory examination may reveal abnormal liver function tests. Alpha-fetoprotein is a specific marker for hepatoma but can also be elevated in embryonic tumors. Radiographic studies are used to differentiate benign and malignant lesions. Ultrasonography can distinguish cystic from solid lesions, whereas CT or

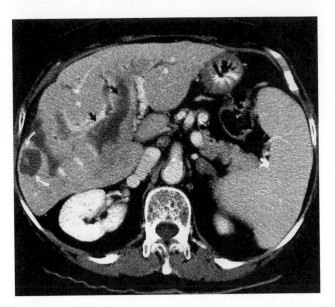

Figure 11-2 • Hepatocellular carcinoma with portal venous thrombosis. CT image demonstrates portal vein thrombus (black arrows on thrombosed right and left portal veins). A mass (curved white arrows) is present in the liver's right lobe.
From Kelsen DP, Daly JM, Kern SE, Levin B, Tepper JE. *Gastrointestinal Oncology: Principles and Practice.* Philadelphia, PA: Lippincott Williams & Wilkins; 2002:10–16.

magnetic resonance imaging (MRI) can reveal multiple lesions and clarify anatomic relationships (Fig. 11-2). Hepatic arteriography can diagnose a hemangioma.

TREATMENT

Treatment involves resection of the tumor. Survival without treatment averages 3 months; resection can extend survival to 3 years, with a 5-year survival of 11% to 46%. The decision to resect the tumor depends on comorbid disease and the location and size of the tumor. When possible, wedge resection should be performed, as formal hepatic lobectomy does not provide any additional survival benefit. Patients with small tumors that are not candidates for resection due to tumor location or concomitant cirrhosis should be considered for liver transplantation.

Metastatic disease occurs in decreasing frequency from lung, colon, pancreas, breast, and stomach. When colon cancer metastasizes to the liver, resection of up to three lesions has been shown to improve survival and should be attempted as long as the operative risk is not prohibitive. In general, liver metastases from other tumors should not be resected.

🔑 11-3 KEY POINTS

1. Hepatocellular carcinoma is extremely common worldwide but relatively rare in the United States.
2. Causes of hepatocellular carcinoma include cirrhosis, aflatoxin, smoking, and vinyl chloride.
3. The prognosis for hepatocellular carcinoma is poor.

LIVER ABSCESSES

ETIOLOGY

Liver abscesses are most frequently due to bacteria, amebas, or the tapeworm *Echinococcus*. Bacterial abscesses usually arise from an intra-abdominal infection in the appendix, gallbladder, or intestine but may be due to trauma or a complication of a surgical procedure. Causative organisms are principally gut flora, including *Escherichia coli*, *Klebsiella*, enterococci, and anaerobes (including *Bacteroides*). Amebic abscesses are an infrequent complication of gastrointestinal amebiasis.

EPIDEMIOLOGY

Pyogenic abscesses are responsible for fewer than 1 in 500 adult hospital admissions. Amebic abscesses occur in 3% to 25% of patients with gastrointestinal amebiasis (Fig. 11-3). Risk factors include human immunodeficiency virus, alcohol abuse, and foreign travel. *Echinococcus* is most commonly seen in eastern Europe, Greece, South Africa, South America, and Australia; although rare in the United States, it is the most common cause of liver abscesses worldwide.

HISTORY

Patients with pyogenic or amebic abscesses usually have nonspecific complaints of vague abdominal pain, weight loss, malaise, anorexia, and fever. Travel to an endemic region may suggest *Echinococcus*.

PHYSICAL EXAMINATION

The liver may be tender or enlarged, and jaundice may occur. Rupture of an abscess can lead to peritonitis, sepsis, and circulatory collapse.

DIAGNOSTIC EVALUATION

The white blood cell count and transaminase levels are elevated. Antibodies to ameba are found in 98% of patients with amebic abscesses but in fewer than 5% of those with pyogenic abscesses. Echinococcal infection produces eosinophilia and a positive heme agglutination test. Ultrasonography is approximately 90% sensitive for demonstrating a lesion; CT is slightly better. The presence of multiple cysts, or "sand," on CT is suggestive of *Echinococcus*. Sampling of the cyst contents with CT or ultrasound guidance reveals the causative organism in the case of pyogenic abscesses but does not usually lead to a diagnosis in amebic abscesses. Aspiration of echinococcal cysts is contraindicated because of the risk of contaminating the peritoneal cavity.

TREATMENT

Pyogenic abscesses require antibiotics alone or in combination with percutaneous or open drainage. Amebic abscesses are treated with metronidazole (Flagyl), with or without chloroquine, and surgical drainage is reserved for complications, including rupture. Echinococcal abscesses require an open procedure. Scolicidal agents (e.g., ethanol or 20% sodium chloride) are instilled directly into the cyst, followed by drainage, with care not to spill the organisms into the peritoneum.

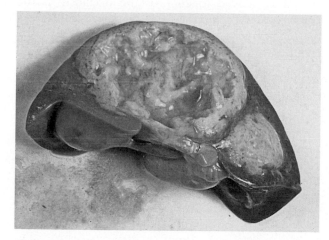

Figure 11-3 • Amebic abscesses of the liver. The cut surface of the liver shows multiple abscesses containing "anchovy paste" material.
From Rubin E, Farber JL. *Pathology*. 3rd ed. Philadelphia, PA: Lippincott Williams & Wilkins; 1999: 9–75.

♠ 11-4 KEY POINT

1. Liver abscesses are most commonly caused by bacteria, amebas, or *Echinococcus*.

PORTAL HYPERTENSION

ETIOLOGY

Portal hypertension is caused by processes that impede hepatic blood flow, either at the presinusoidal, sinusoidal, or postsinusoidal levels. Presinusoidal causes include schistosomiasis and portal vein thrombosis. The principal sinusoidal cause in the United States is cirrhosis, usually caused by alcohol but also by hepatitis B and C. Cirrhosis develops in approximately 15% of alcoholics. Postsinusoidal causes of portal hypertension include Budd-Chiari syndrome (hepatic vein occlusion), pericarditis, and right-sided heart failure.

COMPLICATIONS

Bleeding varices are a life-threatening complication of portal hypertension. When portal pressures rise, flow through the hemorrhoidal, umbilical, or coronary veins becomes the low-resistance route for blood flow. The coronary vein empties into the plexus of veins draining the stomach and esophagus (Fig. 11-4). Engorgement of these veins places the patient at risk of bleeding into the esophagus or stomach.

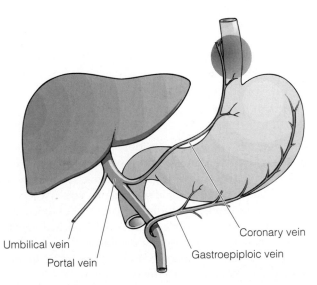

Umbilical vein

Portal vein

Coronary vein

Gastroepiploic vein

Figure 11-4 • Selected collateral circulation in portal hypertension.

HISTORY

Alcoholism, hepatitis, or previous variceal hemorrhages are common.

PHYSICAL EXAMINATION

A variety of physical findings, including ascites, jaundice, "cherubic face," spider angioma, testicular atrophy, gynecomastia, and palmar erythema, may suggest the diagnosis.

DIAGNOSTIC EVALUATION

Laboratory examination may reveal increased liver enzymes, which may return to normal with advanced cirrhosis as the amount of functioning hepatic parenchyma decreases. Tests of liver synthetic function, including clotting times and serum albumin, may be abnormal.

TREATMENT

Patients with portal hypertension are placed on beta-blockers to decrease the risk of bleeding. Endoscopic surveillance and banding are useful in preventing bleeding episodes

For patients with upper gastrointestinal bleeds, large-bore intravenous lines and volume resuscitation should be started immediately. A nasogastric tube should be placed to confirm the diagnosis. If the patient cannot be lavaged clear, suggesting active bleeding, emergency endoscopy is both diagnostic and therapeutic. Endoscopy is greater than 90% effective in controlling acute bleeding from esophageal varices. Should this fail, balloon tamponade with a Sengstaken-Blakemore tube and vasopressin infusion should be considered. Use of the Sengstaken-Blakemore tube involves passing the gastric balloon into the stomach, exerting gentle traction on the tube, and then inflating the esophageal balloon to tamponade bleeding. Although effective in stopping life-threatening hemorrhage, the tube can produce gastric and esophageal ischemia and must be used with extreme caution. Transjugular intrahepatic portosystemic shunting (TIPS) has a high rate of success in controlling acute bleeding and is usually preferred to an emergent surgical shunt, though this is also an option (Fig. 11-5).

Approximately 40% of patients with varices will develop a bleeding complication. Seventy percent of

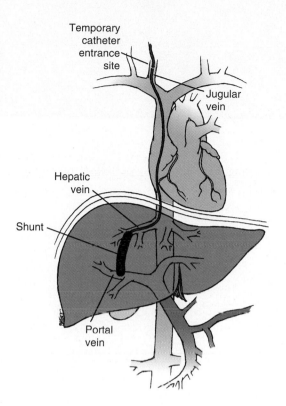

patients with a first episode will rebleed. For this reason, a definitive procedure should be considered after the initial episode is controlled.

11-5 KEY POINTS

1. Portal hypertension has presinusoidal, sinusoidal, and postsinusoidal causes.
2. Variceal hemorrhage is life-threatening, but endoscopy is usually successful in controlling bleeding.
3. Because of the high recurrence rate, a definitive procedure should be considered after the first episode of variceal bleeding.

Figure 11-5 • TIPS. A metallic shunt is placed from the hepatic vein to the right portal vein via a catheter introduced through the internal jugular vein.
From Blackbourne LH. *Advanced Surgical Recall.* 2nd ed. Baltimore, MD: Lippincott Williams & Wilkins; 2004.

References

Llovet JM. Updated treatment approach to hepatocellular carcinoma. *J Gastroenterol.* 2005;40(3):225–235.

Ochs A. Transjugular intrahepatic portosystemic shunt. *Dig Dis.* 2005;23(1):56–64.

BENIGN TUMORS OF THE TRACHEA AND BRONCHI

ANATOMY

The lungs are divided into three lobes and ten segments on the right, and two lobes and nine segments on the left. The decreased number of divisions on the left can be thought of as space taken up by the heart. The right mainstem bronchus forms a gentler curve into the trachea than does the left mainstem bronchus; therefore, aspiration of foreign bodies or gastric contents is more likely to affect the right lung (Fig. 12-1), specifically the dependent portions that are the superior segment of the right lower lobe and the posterior segment of the right upper lobe. Arterial supply to the lungs is through the pulmonary artery as well as the bronchial arteries, which arise from the aorta and intercostal vessels (Fig. 12-2).

PATHOLOGY

Types of benign tumors include squamous papilloma, angioma, fibroma, leiomyoma, and chondroma. Squamous papillomatosis is associated with human papilloma viruses 6 and 11.

EPIDEMIOLOGY

Truly benign neoplasms of the trachea and bronchi are rare.

HISTORY

Patients commonly present with recurrent pneumonias, cough, or hemoptysis.

PHYSICAL EXAMINATION

Patients may have decreased breath sounds on the affected side, with the additional signs and symptoms due to postobstructive pneumonia.

DIAGNOSTIC EVALUATION

Chest radiography may demonstrate a mass, and there is often a postobstructive pneumonia if the lesion significantly narrows the bronchial lumen.

TREATMENT

Angiomas frequently regress, and observation is recommended. Other lesions require surgical removal to relieve symptoms and establish a diagnosis. This may require partial lung resection or sleeve resection, with reanastomosis of a bronchus or the trachea. Squamous papillomatosis has a high recurrence rate.

12-1 KEY POINT

1. Benign lesions of the trachea and bronchi are rare and may require partial lung resection or sleeve resection for treatment.

TUMORS WITH MALIGNANT POTENTIAL

Tumors with malignant potential include bronchial carcinoids, adenoid cystic carcinoma, and mucoepidermoid tumors. Although they do not usually show invasive or metastatic features, a subset of each of

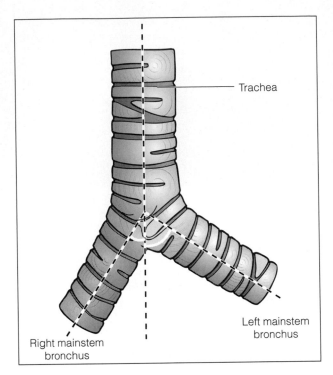

Trachea

Left mainstem bronchus

Right mainstem bronchus

Figure 12-1 • Anatomy of the mainstem bronchi showing asymmetric angulation.

these tumors does. Carcinoid tumors, which are malignant in approximately 10% of patients, may cause paraneoplastic syndromes through release of various substances, including histamine, serotonin, vasoactive intestinal peptide, gastrin, growth hormone, insulin, glucagon, and catecholamines.

EPIDEMIOLOGY

These tumors make up fewer than 5% of all pulmonary neoplasms and have no obvious age or sex predilection. Carcinoids make up approximately 1% of all lung tumors; adenoid cystic carcinoma, approximately 0.5%; and mucoepidermoid, approximately 0.2%.

HISTORY

Patients most commonly complain of cough, dyspnea, hemoptysis, or recurrent pneumonia. Less frequently, carcinoid tumors may produce carcinoid syndrome, with complaints of flushing and diarrhea, as well as manifestations of specific hormone excess. This syndrome only occurs in approximately 3% of patients with carcinoid tumors.

PHYSICAL EXAMINATION

The patient may have respiratory compromise or decreased breath sounds. Carcinoid tumors may cause valvular heart disease with signs of pulmonic stenosis or tricuspid regurgitation.

DIAGNOSTIC EVALUATION

Chest radiography may reveal a lesion or postobstructive pneumonia. Bronchoscopy is useful to obtain tissue diagnosis and define bronchial anatomy. Computed tomography (CT) of the chest is routine for preoperative planning.

TREATMENT

These tumors should all be resected. Long-term survival for carcinoid tumors is 80%; for adenoid cystic carcinoma and mucoepidermoid tumors, the prognosis is also favorable.

🔑 12-2 KEY POINT

1. Carcinoid tumors can release a variety of substances, causing paraneoplastic syndromes.

LUNG CANCER

EPIDEMIOLOGY

Lung cancer is the leading cause of cancer-related death for both men and women in North America, responsible for more than 150,000 deaths each year in the United States and accounting for almost 30% of all cancer deaths. More than 80% of lung cancers are smoking related. In the United States, more people die each year from lung cancer than from breast, prostate, and colorectal cancers combined. Lung cancer kills more men than does prostate cancer and more women than breast cancer. Lung cancer incidence rates among women continue to rise; deaths from lung cancer in women have increased 400% between 1960 and 1990. Smoking cessation significantly reduces an individual's risk of developing lung cancer, although the level of risk remains greater than for nonsmokers. Asbestos, formaldehyde, radon gas,

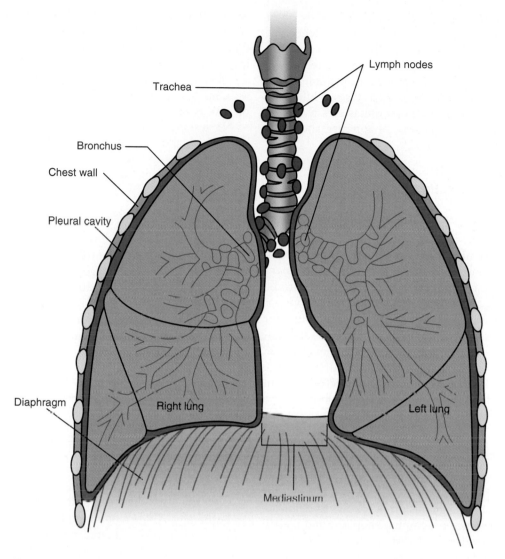

Figure 12-2 • Anatomy of the lungs.

arsenic, uranium, chromates, and nickel have been identified as carcinogens, especially when combined with smoking.

PATHOLOGY

Lung cancer is divided into small cell (20–25%) and non–small cell carcinoma (75–80%). Nonsmall cell carcinoma is further divided into squamous cell carcinoma (30%), adenocarcinoma (35%), and large cell carcinoma (10%). Small cell cancer is usually centrally located and may be associated with paraneoplastic syndromes. Approximately 5% of patients have symptoms of inappropriate secretion of antidiuretic

hormone, whereas 3% to 5% have Cushing syndrome from adrenocorticotropin (ACTH) production. Squamous cell cancer usually occurs centrally and can be associated with symptoms of hypercalcemia secondary to production of a substance similar to parathyroid hormone. Adenocarcinoma typically occurs at the periphery.

HISTORY

Most patients come to medical attention due to signs and symptoms indicating advanced disease. Ninety percent of patients with lung cancer are symptomatic at the time of diagnosis. Worsening cough with increased sputum production and hemoptysis often indicates airway obstruction by tumor. Recurrent pneumonia requiring antibiotic therapy is common. Persistent chest, back, or shoulder pain is related to nerve involvement or direct tumor invasion. Bone pain indicates distant skeletal metastases, while neurologic symptoms indicate brain metastases. Systemic symptoms include fatigue, loss of appetite, and unintentional weight loss.

PHYSICAL EXAMINATION

Chest auscultation may reveal diminished breath sounds due to pneumonia or malignant pleural effusion. Supraclavicular lymphadenopathy may be present. Recent onset of hoarseness indicates involvement of the recurrent laryngeal nerve. Horner syndrome (ptosis, myosis, and anhydrosis) results from a superior sulcus tumor causing neural compression. Superior vena cava syndrome and Pancoast syndrome (shoulder and arm pain on the affected side) may occur. Paralysis of the diaphragm indicates phrenic nerve involvement. Patients with advanced disease are usually sickly and exhibit significant weight loss.

DIAGNOSTIC EVALUATION

Chest x-ray is often the modality first used to diagnose a suspicious pulmonary lesion. Chest CT including the liver and adrenal glands often follows to delineate tumor size, presence of lymphadenopathy and pleural effusion, and evidence of distant disease. Bone scan and brain imaging may also be obtained, if necessary. Noninvasive functional testing for distant disease can be done by positron emission tomography (PET) scan. This information allows for clinical staging.

Invasive testing is usually required for definitive diagnosis. Flexible bronchoscopy allows for tissue biopsy and bronchial washings. Transthoracic CT-guided fine-needle biopsy can also provide diagnostic tissue sampling. Mediastinoscopy with lymph node biopsy can be diagnostic while also providing information for accurate staging.

STAGING

The TNM (tumor, nodes, metastases) system is used (Table 12-1). T1 lesions are less than 3 cm; T2 lesions are greater than 3 cm or involve the main bronchus greater than 2 cm from the carina or involve the visceral pleura. T3 lesions invade the chest wall, diaphragm, mediastinal pleura, or pericardium or involve the main bronchus within 2 cm of the carina. T4 lesions invade the heart, great vessels, mediastinum, trachea, esophagus, vertebral bodies, or carina or have malignant effusions or satellite tumors.

N1 lesions have positive nodes in the ipsilateral peribronchial or hilar region. N2 lesions have positive nodes in the ipsilateral mediastinal or subcarinal region. N3 lesions have metastases either to contralateral nodes or ipsilateral scalene or supraclavicular regions.

Stage IA lesions are T1, N0, M0 lesions. Stage IB lesions are T2, N0, M0 lesions. Stage IIA lesions are T1, N1, M0 lesions. Stage IIB lesions are T2, N1, M0 or T3, N0, M0 lesions. Stage IIIA lesions are T3, N1, M0; T1, N2, M0; T2, N2, M0; or T3, N2, M0 lesions. Stage IIIB lesions are tumors without distant metastases, including primary tumors to T4 and N3 regional lymph node metastases. Stage IV patients have evidence of distant metastases.

TREATMENT

Small cell lung cancer is usually widely disseminated at the time of diagnosis, so surgery is rarely indicated. Only very early stage tumors are considered potentially resectable. The standard treatment for this aggressive disease is chemotherapy—usually combination therapy with cisplatin and etoposide and radiotherapy. Triplet combination chemotherapy is often used, as is accelerated radiotherapy. If patients have favorable treatment responses and exhibit complete remission, then prophylactic whole-brain radiation is recommended to decrease the chance of cerebral metastases (50% of untreated patients develop brain metastases).

Non–small cell lung cancer treatment is based on clinical stage as well. For early-stage cancer (stage I and II, as well as highly selected stage III lesions), surgery followed by chemotherapy is standard care. The most common procedure performed is lobectomy.

Results of recent clinical trials now support the use of chemotherapy in all patients with completely resected lung cancer. Standard chemotherapy regimens include a platinum agent (cisplatin or carboplatin) and a nonplatinum agent (etoposide, irinotecan, paclitaxel, gemcitabine, and others). Radiotherapy is often used if mediastinal lymph nodes are involved (stage III).

■ **TABLE 12-1** Current International Staging System for Non–Small Cell Lung Cancer

Staging	
Primary tumor (T)	
TX	Tumor proved by the presence of malignant cells in bronchopulmonary secretions but not visualized roentgenographically or bronchoscopically, or any tumor that cannot be assessed as in a retreatment staging.
T0	No evidence of primary tumor
Tis	Carcinoma in situ
T1*	A tumor that is 3 cm or less in greatest dimension, surrounded by lung or visceral pleura, and without evidence of invasion proximal to a lobar bronchus at bronchoscopy
T2	A tumor more than 3 cm in greatest dimension, or a tumor of any size that either invades the visceral pleura or has associated atelectasis or obstructive pneumonitis extending to the hilar region (At bronchoscopy, the proximal extent of demonstrable tumor must be within a lobar bronchus or at least 2 cm distal to the carina. Any associated atelectasis or obstructive pneumonitis must involve less than an entire lung.)
T3	A tumor of any size with direct extension into the chest wall (including superior sulcus tumors), diaphragm, or the mediastinal pleura or pericardium without involving the heart, great vessels, trachea, esophagus, or vertebral body, or a tumor in the main bronchus within 2 cm of the carina without involving the carina
T4**	A tumor of any size with invasion of the mediastinum or involving the heart, great vessels, trachea, esophagus, vertebral body, or carina or presence of malignant pleural effusion
Nodal involvement (N)	
N0	No demonstrable metastasis to regional lymph nodes
N1	Metastasis to lymph nodes in the peribronchial or the ipsilateral hilar region, or both, including direct extension
N2	Metastasis to ipsilateral mediastinal lymph nodes and subcarinal lymph nodes
N3	Metastasis to contralateral mediastinal lymph nodes, contralateral hilar lymph nodes, ipsilateral or contralateral scalene lymph nodes, or supraclavicular lymph nodes
Distant metastasis (M)	
M0	No (known) distant metastasis
M1	Distant metastasis present—specify sites
Stage grouping	
Occult carcinoma	TX, N0, M0
Stage 0	Tis, carcinoma in situ
Stage I	T1, N0, M0
	T2, N0, M0
Stage II	T1, N1, M0
	T2, N1, M0
Stage IIIa	T3, N0, M0
	T3, N1, M0
	T1–3, N2, M0

(Continued)

■ TABLE 12-1 Current International Staging System for Non–Small Cell Lung Cancer *(continued)*	
Staging	
Stage IIIb	Any T, N3, M0
	T4, any N, M0
Stage IV	Any T, any N, M1

* The uncommon superficial tumor of any size with its invasive component limited to the bronchial wall that may extend proximal to the main bronchus is classified as T1.

** Most pleural effusions associated with lung cancer are due to tumor. There are, however, a few patients in whom cytopathologic examination of pleural fluid (on more than one specimen) is negative for tumor and in whom the fluid is nonbloody and is not an exudate. In cases in which these elements and clinical judgment dictate that the effusion is not related to the tumor, the patient should be staged T1, T2, or T3, excluding effusion as a staging element.

PROGNOSIS

Lung cancer remains a lethal disease, despite recent advances. The 5-year survival rate for all patients is just over 10%. For early-stage asymptomatic non–small cell lung cancers (stage IA), usually detected incidentally on chest radiograph, the 5-year survival rate is approximately 80%. This figure rapidly drops to 55% for stage IB and to 30% for stage II disease. Given the overall poor survival figures, there has been a resurgence of interest in screening tests using spiral CT scans for early detection of lung cancer. This is an active area of ongoing research.

Long-term survival in small cell lung cancer is rare.

🔑 12-3 KEY POINTS

1. Lung cancer is the leading cause of cancer-related death in North America.
2. More than 80% of lung cancers are smoking related.
3. Most patients are symptomatic at the time of presentation and are not surgical candidates.
4. Accurate preoperative staging is required to determine appropriate treatment.
5. Early-stage lung cancer is treated with surgery and chemotherapy.
6. Overall, prognosis is poor.

MESOTHELIOMA

PATHOLOGY

Mesothelioma is a malignant lesion derived most commonly from the visceral pleura.

EPIDEMIOLOGY

The tumor is rare. Asbestos is the major risk factor. Cigarette smoking markedly increases the incidence of mesothelioma in patients exposed to asbestos.

HISTORY

Chest pain from local extension, dyspnea secondary to pleural effusion, weight loss, and unexplained night sweats may occur.

PHYSICAL EXAMINATION

The patient may have decreased breath sounds on the side of the tumor due to pleural effusion and long entrapment.

DIAGNOSTIC EVALUATION

Chest radiography often demonstrates a pleural effusion. Thoracocentesis typically yields bloody fluid, and cytology is often negative for malignant disease. Patients with a suggestive history and a recurrent pleural effusion with no clear etiology should undergo thoracoscopy and pleural biopsy, even in the presence of negative fluid cytology.

TREATMENT

Overall prognosis is poor, with few survivors living beyond 2 years. Early-stage lesions may be resectable but require induction chemotherapy followed by extrapleural pneumonectomy, a significantly morbid procedure. Chemotherapy and radiotherapy are used for nonoperative candidates.

PNEUMOTHORAX

The lung is covered by visceral pleura, and the inner chest wall is covered by parietal pleura. These two continuous surfaces form a potential space. Simple pneumothorax occurs when air enters this space and the lung falls away from the chest wall (Fig. 12-3). Open pneumothorax occurs when a defect in the chest wall allows continuous entry of air from the outside. Tension pneumothorax occurs when air enters the potential space but cannot escape. A valvelike effect allows pressure to increase, thereby forcibly collapsing the ipsilateral lung and compressing mediastinal structures.

ETIOLOGY

Spontaneous pneumothorax usually occurs in young thin males or in older patients with bullous emphysema. It can also occur in patients on mechanical ventilation, especially if high inspiratory pressures are required. Infection, specifically tuberculosis or *Pneumocystis carinii*, can cause pneumothorax, as can lung tumors. Placement of central venous catheters results in pneumothorax in 1% of cases. Thoracocentesis, needle biopsy, and operative trauma are other iatrogenic causes. Open pneumothorax is caused by trauma, whereas tension pneumothorax can occur by any of the above mechanisms.

HISTORY

Patients can be entirely asymptomatic, or they may complain of dyspnea or pleuritic chest pain.

PHYSICAL EXAMINATION

Simple pneumothorax may result in decreased breath sounds and hyperresonance on the affected side. Tension pneumothorax may cause tachycardia, hypotension, and hypoxia, and the trachea may be displaced away from the affected side.

DIAGNOSTIC EVALUATION

Chest radiography reveals absence of lung markings in the affected area, usually in the apex, in an upright film. A visible line corresponding to the visceral pleural surface of the lung is evident. Tracheal deviation or mediastinal shift suggests tension pneumothorax.

TREATMENT

Simple pneumothoraxes of less than 20% can be observed if no increase in size is demonstrated on serial chest x-rays. Indications for chest tube replacement include those with size greater than 20% or those that increase in size during observation. Open pneumothorax requires repair of the defect and tube thoracostomy. Symptomatic tension pneumothorax is a surgical emergency and requires immediate needle thoracostomy, usually in the midclavicular line in the second intercostal space on the affected side. This will decompress the chest and allow normalization of hemodynamics and oxygenation. Tube thoracostomy should then follow.

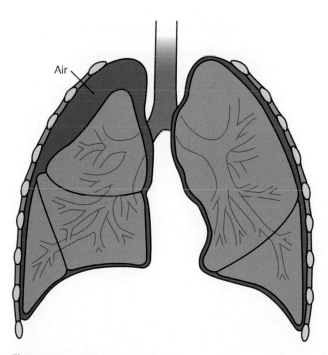

Air

Figure 12-3 • Right pneumothorax.

EMPYEMA

Empyema is an infection within the pleural space.

ETIOLOGY

Empyema is most commonly caused by pneumonia, lung abscess, a postoperative complication of thoracic surgery, or esophageal perforation. The most common organisms are those that cause primary lung infection, including *Staphylococcus, Streptococcus, Pseudomonas, Klebsiella, Escherichia coli, Proteus,* and *Bacteroides.*

HISTORY

The patient may have a history of previous pneumonia, thoracic surgery, or esophageal instrumentation. Fatigue, lethargy, and shaking chills may occur.

PHYSICAL EXAMINATION

The patient is often systemically ill. Fever and decreased breath sounds at the affected lung base are common.

DIAGNOSTIC EVALUATION

The serum white blood cell count is elevated. Chest radiography reveals a pleural effusion. Aspiration of the pleural fluid by thoracentesis shows an exudative effusion, characterized by a high white blood cell count with predominantly polymorphonuclear cells, a low pH, a low glucose, and high lactic dehydrogenase (LDH). Bacteria on Gram stain and culture may be present.

TREATMENT

On rare occasions, antibiotics and needle aspiration alone are successful, but usually tube thoracostomy is required.

12-6 KEY POINT

1. Empyema is usually treated with tube thoracostomy and antibiotics.

References

Baas P, Van Ruty S, Zoetmulder FA. Surgical treatment of malignant pleural mesothelioma: a review. *Chest.* 2003;123(2):551–561.

Jantz MA, Pierson DJ. Pneumothorax and barotrauma. *Clin Chest Med.* 1994;15(1):75–91.

Mitchell C, Mitchell G. Lung cancer. *Aust Fam Physician.* 2004;33(5):321–325.

Prostate and Male Reproductive Organs

BENIGN PROSTATIC HYPERPLASIA

Benign prostatic hyperplasia (BPH) is a common condition of the prostate gland seen in older men. BPH is clinically important because it is the most common cause of urinary outlet obstruction in men over 50 years of age. Untreated, this results in stasis, which increases the risk of urinary tract infection and bladder stones. Over time, bladder decompensation can result in chronic urinary retention with overflow or renal failure secondary to high-pressure urinary retention.

PATHOGENESIS

Prostate gland growth is influenced by steroid hormones. However, the exact mechanism of prostatic hyperplasia remains unclear. Interestingly, BPH does not occur in castrated men or pseudohermaphrodites, both of whom lack dihydrotestosterone (DHT), the active metabolite of testosterone. Estrogens have also been implicated in prostatic hyperplasia, because in aging men, the levels of estrogens rise and those of androgens fall.

The specific area of cellular hyperplasia is the transitional zone or periurethral area of the prostate. The periurethral glandular elements undergo hyperplasia, causing an increase in glandular mass that results in compression of the prostatic urethra and the onset of obstructive symptoms (Fig. 13-1).

EPIDEMIOLOGY

The prevalence of BPH increases with age. Autopsy studies show that at least 50% of men over the age of 50 have significant enlargement of the prostate due to BPH. Rarely does a patient present before age 50, because the doubling time of the hyperplastic gland is slow. By age 90, roughly 90% of males have a significant degree of hyperplasia. All men with intact functional testes are at risk for development of BPH.

CLINICAL MANIFESTATIONS

History

Any older man presenting with obstructive urinary symptoms must be suspected of having BPH. Symptoms include urinary hesitancy, intermittency, decreased force of urinary stream, and a sensation of incomplete bladder emptying after voiding. Secondary symptoms are a consequence of urinary stasis. High postvoid residual volumes promote bacterial growth, leading to urinary tract infection. Stasis can also promote the formation of bladder calculi. Most seriously, high-pressure chronic retention can cause bilateral hydroureteronephrosis and subsequent renal failure.

Physical Examination

A careful rectal examination reveals an enlarged symmetric rubbery gland. The size of the gland has no relationship to symptomatology. A small gland may produce a high degree of outflow obstruction, whereas a large gland may produce no symptoms at all. The suprapubic region should be palpated to rule out a grossly distended bladder.

Diagnostic Evaluation

Urine should be obtained for sediment analysis and microbiologic cultures. Serum blood urea nitrogen and creatinine levels should be checked for evidence of

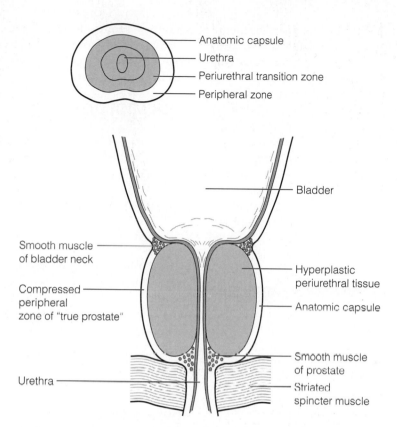

Anatomic capsule
Urethra
Periurethral transition zone
Peripheral zone

Bladder

Smooth muscle
of bladder neck

Compressed
peripheral
zone of "true prostate"

Urethra

Hyperplastic
periurethral tissue

Anatomic capsule

Smooth muscle
of prostate

Striated
spincter muscle

Figure 13-1 • Benign prostatic hyperplasia causing urethral compression.
The enlarged periurethral glands are enclosed by the orange peel–like sur
gical capsule, which is composed of compressed true prostatic tissue.

renal insufficiency. If chronic urinary retention is suspected, a postvoid residual can be checked by straight catheterization or bladder ultrasonography. Urinary flow rate is assessed by measuring the volume of urine voided during a 5-second period. A flow rate of <50 mL in 5 seconds is evidence of bladder outlet obstruction. Ultrasonography, intravenous pyelography (IVP), or computed tomographic (CT) scan can be used for imaging the urinary tract. Information regarding size of the prostate, presence of bladder stones, the postvoid residual volume, and hydronephrosis can be obtained. Transrectal ultrasonography is used to evaluate either an irregular prostate when found on examination or an elevated prostate-specific antigen (PSA) level.

Treatment

The goals of drug therapy for BPH are to relax smooth muscle in the prostate and bladder neck or to induce regression of cellular hyperplasia, thereby enhancing urinary outflow from the bladder to the urethra. Alpha

blockade of adrenergic receptors produces smooth muscle relaxation of both prostate and bladder neck. An infrequent side effect of alpha-antagonists (e.g., terazosin) is postural hypotension (2%–8%). Prostatic hyperplasia can also be treated with 5-alpha reductase inhibitors (e.g., finasteride), which block the conversion of testosterone to DHT without lowering serum levels of circulation testosterone. However, the effectiveness of 5-alpha reductase inhibitors is less than half that seen with alpha-blockers.

Surgical relief of obstruction is necessary when medical therapy fails. The indications for surgery are a postvoid residual volume >100 mL, acute urinary retention, chronic urinary retention with overflow dribbling, gross hematuria on more than one occasion, and recurrent urinary tract infections. Additional indications are patient request for restoration of normal voiding pattern because of excessive nocturia or dribbling.

The procedure of choice is transurethral resection of the prostate (TURP). With the patient in the lithotomy position, the resectoscope is introduced via the urethra into the bladder. The occlusive prostate tissue is identified, and under direct vision, the tissue is shaved away using an electrified wire loop. Extravasated blood and tissue fragments are evacuated as the bladder is continuously irrigated with a nonelectrolytic isotonic solution. An indwelling catheter is left in place for 1 to 7 days. To minimize the blood loss and side effects of the standard TURP technique, alternative minimally invasive outpatient procedures have been developed and are applicable to select patients. Transurethral needle ablation (TUNA) and focused ultrasound—both of which are less invasive modalities than TURP—ablate prostate tissue by locally heating the tissue. Although these procedures have excellent short-term results in selected patients, long-term efficacy is not well established.

🔑 13-1 KEY POINTS

1. Benign prostatic hyperplasia (BPH) is a disease of older men that causes bladder outlet obstruction.
2. Obstructive urinary symptoms include hesitancy, poor stream, incomplete bladder emptying, nocturia, and dribbling.
3. Secondary symptoms arising from urinary stasis include urinary tract infections, bladder calculi, hydroureteronephrosis, and renal failure.
4. BPH is medically treated by alpha blockade to relax prostate and bladder neck smooth muscle and occasionally by 5-alpha reductase inhibition to block dihydrotestosterone production and cause regression of cellular hyperplasia.
5. BPH is surgically treated by transurethral resection of the prostate and other techniques.

PROSTATE CANCER

Prostate cancer is the most common malignancy of the male genitourinary (GU) tract. Indolent tumor growth and a long latency period account for the majority of cases (~80%) being clinically silent. Most prostate cancers are only discovered on postmortem examination. Management and prognosis depend on stage of tumor.

PATHOGENESIS

The vast majority of prostate cancer (~95%) is adenocarcinoma. Tumors arise from the glandular epithelium in the peripheral zone of the prostate. Tumor growth is hormonally influenced, as testosterone exerts a stimulatory effect while estrogens and antiandrogens are inhibitory. Tumors are histologically graded using the Gleason grading system, with scores from 2 (well differentiated) to 10 (poorly differentiated). Tumor grade correlates with prognosis.

EPIDEMIOLOGY

Prostate cancer is a malignancy of older men, usually occurring after age 60. The disease is more common in black men than in white.

CLINICAL MANIFESTATIONS

History

Early prostate cancer is usually asymptomatic and is typically only detected on screening examination. Many patients present with evidence of obstructive symptoms indicating invasion or compression (poor stream, incomplete bladder emptying, nocturia). Such patients are commonly misdiagnosed as having BPH. Metastatic disease is often manifested by bony pain or ureteric obstruction.

Physical Examination

Digital rectal examination and PSA measurement are the principal methods of screening. Tumor staging is based on the degree of spread: T1–T2 is localized spread within the prostate, T3–T4 is local spread to seminal vesicles or pelvic wall, and M1 indicates metastatic disease. Pattern of spread is via lymphatics to iliac and periaortic nodes and via the circulation to bone, lung, and liver.

Diagnosis

As for most cancers, prostate cancer requires tissue diagnosis. Typically, a hard nodule is detected on digital rectal examination and a follow-up transrectal ultrasound is obtained for needle biopsy of the prostate. The procedure is well tolerated and performed on an outpatient basis.

Chest x-ray is performed to evaluate for lung metastases. Liver function tests may detect liver metastases. If bone metastases are suspected based on presenting symptoms, a bone scan is indicated.

Treatment

Treatment for prostate cancer is based on the stage and grade of the tumor. Two common staging systems are the Gleason score and the TNM stage (Tables 13-1 and 13-2). The treatment options for localized disease

<table>
<tr><td colspan="2">■ **TABLE 13-1** Gleason Score</td></tr>
</table>

2–4	Well-differentiated tumors with cells that are expected to grow slowly and not spread readily
5–7	Moderately differentiated tumor cells
8–10	Poorly differentiated tumors with cells that are likely to grow rapidly and spread to other parts of the body (metastasize)

(T1–T2) include radical prostatectomy, external-beam radiotherapy, or interstitial irradiation with implants. For local spread (T3–T4), the treatment is external-beam radiotherapy, with the addition of hormonal therapy for more advanced cases. Treatment for metastatic disease is hormonal ablation, as most prostate cancers are androgen sensitive. Methods of androgen ablation include surgical and pharmacologic options. Bilateral surgical orchiectomy is the gold standard for ablating testosterone production. Chemical castration using

■ TABLE 13-2 AJCC Classification for Prostate Cancer

TNM definitions

Primary tumor (T)

TX	Primary tumor cannot be assessed
T0	No evidence of primary tumor
T1	Clinically inapparent tumor not palpable or visible by imaging
T1a	Tumor incidental histologic finding in ≤5% of tissue resected
T1b	Tumor incidental histologic finding in >5% of tissue resected
T1c	Tumor identified by needle biopsy (e.g., because of elevated PSA)
T2*	Tumor confined within prostate
T2a	Tumor involves 50% of ≤1 lobe or less
T2b	Tumor involves >50% of 1 lobe but not both lobes
T2c	Tumor involves both lobes
T3**	Tumor extends through the prostate capsule
T3a	Extracapsular extension (unilateral or bilateral)
T3b	Tumor invades seminal vesicle(s)
T4	Tumor is fixed or invades adjacent structures other than seminal vesicles: bladder neck, external sphincter, rectum, levator muscles, and/or pelvic wall

PSA, prostate-specific antigen.

* Tumor that is found in one or both lobes by needle biopsy, but that is not palpable or reliably visible by imaging, is classified as T1c.

** Invasion into the prostatic apex or into (but not beyond) the prostatic capsule is not classified as T3, but as T2.

Regional lymph nodes (N)

Regional lymph nodes are the nodes of the true pelvis, which essentially are the pelvic nodes below the bifurcation of the common iliac arteries. They include the following groups (laterality does not affect the N classification): pelvic (not otherwise specified [NOS]), hypogastric, obturator, iliac (i.e., internal, external, NOS), and sacral (lateral, presacral, promontory [e.g., Gerotas], or NOS). Distant lymph nodes are outside the confines of the true pelvis. They can be imaged using ultrasound, computed tomography, magnetic resonance imaging, or lymphangiography, and include: aortic (para-aortic, periaortic, or lumbar), common iliac, inguinal (deep), superficial inguinal (femoral), supraclavicular, cervical, scalene, and retroperitoneal (NOS) nodes. Although enlarged lymph nodes can occasionally be visualized, because of a stage migration associated with PSA screening, very few patients will be found to have nodal disease, so false-positive and false-negative results are common when imaging tests are employed. In lieu of imaging, risk tables are usually used to determine individual patient risk of nodal involvement. Involvement of distant lymph nodes is classified as M1a.

(Continued)

TABLE 13-2 AJCC Classification for Prostate Cancer *(continued)*

NX	Regional lymph nodes were not assessed
N0	No regional lymph node metastasis
N1	Metastasis in regional lymph node(s)

Distant metastasis (M)*

MX	Distant metastasis cannot be assessed (not evaluated by any modality)
M0	No distant metastasis
M1	Distant metastasis
M1a	Nonregional lymph node(s)
M1b	Bone(s)
M1c	Other site(s) with or without bone disease

* When more than one site of metastasis is present, the most advanced category (pM1c) is used.

Histopathologic grade (G)

GX	Grade cannot be assessed
G1	Well-differentiated (slight anaplasia) (Gleason 2–4)
G2	Moderately differentiated (moderate anaplasia) (Gleason 5–6)
G3–G4	Poorly differentiated or undifferentiated (marked anaplasia) (Gleason 7–10)

AJCC stage groupings

Stage I

T1a, N0, M0, G1

Stage II

T1a, N0, M0, G2–G4

T1b, N0, M0, any G

T1c, N0, M0, any G

T1, N0, M0, any G

T2, N0, M0, any G

Stage III

T3, N0, M0, any G

Stage IV

T4, N0, M0, any G

Any T, N1, M0, any G

Any T, any N, M1, any G

Jewett staging system

Stage A

Stage A is a clinically undetectable tumor confined to the prostate gland and is an incidental finding at prostatic surgery.

Substage A1	Well-differentiated with focal involvement, usually left untreated
Substage A2	Moderately or poorly differentiated or involves multiple foci in the gland

(Continued)

■ **TABLE 13-2** AJCC Classification for Prostate Cancer *(continued)*

Stage B

Stage B is a tumor confined to the prostate gland.

Substage B0	Nonpalpable, PSA-detected
Substage B1	Single nodule in one lobe of the prostate
Substage B2	More extensive involvement of one lobe or involvement of both lobes

Stage C

Stage C is a tumor clinically localized to the periprostatic area but extending through the prostatic capsule; seminal vesicles may be involved.

Substage C1	Clinical extracapsular extension
Substage C2	Extracapsular tumor producing bladder outlet or ureteral obstruction

Stage D

Stage D is metastatic disease.

Substage D0	Clinically localized disease (prostate only) but persistently elevated enzymatic serum acid phosphatase titers
Substage D1	Regional lymph nodes only
Substage D2	Distant lymph nodes, metastases to bone or visceral organs
Substage D3	D2 prostate cancer patients who relapsed after adequate endocrine therapy

Used with the permission of the American Joint Committee on Cancer (AJCC), Chicago, Illinois. The original source for this material is the AJCC Cancer Staging Manual, 6th ed (2002), published by Springer-Verlag, New York, NY; www.springeronline.com.

luteinizing hormone-releasing hormone (LH-RH) agonists in conjunction with antiandrogens, such as flutamide and cyproterone, produces castrate levels of testosterone. Randomized trials demonstrate that patients with hormone-refractory prostate cancer benefit from docetaxel-based chemotherapy.

13-2 KEY POINTS

1. Prostate cancer is the most common male genitourinary tract malignancy, occurring in older men.
2. Adenocarcinoma arises from glandular epithelium in the periphery of the prostate.
3. Gleason tissue grading (2–10) is used to grade tumor differentiation.
4. Staging is based on the degree of spread: localized, local, or metastatic patterns.
5. Digital rectal examination and prostate-specific antigen measurement are used for prostate cancer screening.
6. Management depends on tumor stage. Treatment options include surgery, radiotherapy, and hormonal ablation.

TESTES

Disorders of the testes requiring surgical management include congenital abnormalities, tumors, and, in the emergent setting, testicular torsion.

CONGENITAL ABNORMALITIES

Cryptorchidism

Cryptorchidism is the failure of normal testicular descent during embryologic development. The cause of failed descent is unknown but may be due to a selective hormone deficiency, gubernaculum abnormality, or intrinsic testicular defect. Such cryptorchid testes fail in spermatogenic function, but they may retain the ability to secrete androgens. The major risk of cryptorchid testes is the increased risk of testes cancer (35–48 times more common than in descended testes). Inguinal hernia is also found in at least 25% of patients with cryptorchidism.

Physical Examination

The testicle remains within the abdomen and cannot be palpated on physical examination.

Treatment

Because spermatogenic failure is progressive, surgical exploration and scrotal placement of the testis should be performed before 2 years of age. If placement of the testicle into the scrotum is not possible, orchiectomy is indicated, because the incidence of cancer of abdominal testes is very high.

Incomplete Descent of the Testis

Incomplete descent of the testis implies a testicle arrested at some point in the path of normal descent but palpable on physical examination. Such testes are usually located within the inguinal canal between the deep and superficial rings. Incompletely descended testes are often associated with congenital indirect hernias due to the incomplete obliteration of the processus vaginalis.

Treatment

Because testicular function is less compromised than in a cryptorchid testicle, the usual treatment is repositioning and orchiopexy within the scrotum. If present, an indirect hernia is repaired concurrently.

Testicular Tumors

Tumors of the testicle are the most common GU malignancy among young men between the ages of 20 and 35. Virtually all neoplasms of the testicle are malignant. Tumors are divided into either germ cell or non–germ cell tumors, depending on their cellular origin. Germ cell tumors predominate, accounting for 90% to 95% of all tumors.

Pathology

Non–germ cell tumors, which arise from Leydig and Sertoli cells, produce excess quantities of androgenizing hormones. Germ cell tumors arise from totipotential cells of the seminiferous tubules. Germ cell tumors are divided into two categories: seminomas and nonseminomatous germ cell tumors (NSGCTs). Seminomas are relatively slow growing and exhibit late invasion. They are usually discovered and surgically removed before metastasis can occur. NSGCTs exhibit greater malignant behavior and metastasize earlier. NSGCTs consist of embryonal (20%), teratoma (5%), choriocarcinoma (<1%), or mixed cell type (40%). Choriocarcinomas are fortunately rare subtypes but are highly invasive, aggressive tumors that metastasize via lymphatic and venous systems early in the disease.

Epidemiology

Seminomas are the most common malignant germ cell tumor. Embryonal carcinoma is usually seen in younger males during childhood. Non–germ cell tumors are relatively rare.

History

Tumors usually manifest as firm, painless testicular masses. Occasionally, the mass may cause a dull ache. Hemorrhage into necrotic tumor or after minor trauma may cause the acute onset of pain. Approximately 10% of patients with testicular tumors have a history of cryptorchidism. Because of excess androgen production, non–germ cell tumors can cause precocious puberty and virilism in young males and impotence and gynecomastia in adults.

Diagnostic Evaluation

Immediate evaluation should include serum for tumor markers (alpha-fetoprotein [AFP], beta-human chorionic gonadotropin [β-hCG]), serum lactic dehydrogenase (LDH), and ultrasound. Tumor markers are not always helpful because seminomas, the most common testicular neoplasm, are usually negative for both AFP and β-hCG. In neoplasms with tumor markers, the level of tumor burden directly relates to AFP/β-hCG levels that can be followed during the postoperative period to evaluate the efficacy of treatment and to detect recurrence.

Treatment

Initial treatment is always radical orchiectomy. Subsequent therapy depends on tumor type, grade, and staging. Retroperitoneal lymph node dissection (RPLND) is standard therapy for stage 1 and 2 NSGCT.

Seminomas are usually highly radiosensitive. Adjuvant treatment with radiation and chemotherapy yields high 5-year survival rates for both localized and metastatic disease.

Torsion of the Spermatic Cord

Torsion of the spermatic cord is a urologic emergency because complete strangulation of the testicular blood supply renders the testicle surgically unsalvageable after approximately 6 hours.

Pathogenesis

Torsion results from an abnormally high attachment of the tunica vaginalis around the distal end of the spermatic cord. This abnormality allows the testis to hang within the tunica compartment, like a bell clapper within a bell—hence the name bell clapper deformity. As such, the testicle is free to twist on its own blood supply, causing pain and ischemic strangulation (Fig. 13-2).

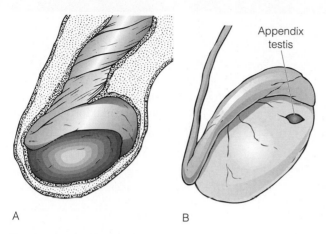

Appendix testis

A   B

Figure 13-2 • Torsion of the testes (A) is the result of twisting of the spermatic cord, usually within the tunica vaginalis; the appendix testis may also become twisted (B).

History

Torsion is usually seen in young males, who present complaining of the rapid onset of severe testicle pain followed by testicle swelling.

Physical examination reveals a high-riding, swollen, tender testicle, oriented horizontally in the scrotum. Pain is worse with elevation of the testes, and the cremasteric reflex is often absent.

Diagnostic Evaluation

A color-flow Doppler ultrasound should be obtained to evaluate for blood flow within the testicle. Absence of flow confirms the diagnosis.

Differential Diagnosis

The differential diagnosis of an acutely swollen, tender testicle includes essentially two diagnoses: torsion of the spermatic cord and advanced epididymitis. Because one can mimic the other, it is vitally important to arrive at a timely diagnosis. Other less common diagnoses include torsion of an appendix testis or appendix epididymis (Fig. 13-2).

Treatment

Prompt surgical exploration and orchiopexy are required to save the testicle from undergoing ischemic necrosis. Because the bell clapper deformity is usually bilateral, orchiopexy of the contralateral testicle is performed concurrently. If the diagnosis is unclear, surgical exploration is required, because an uncorrected torsion will cause necrosis of the testicle.

🔑 13-3 KEY POINTS

1. Cryptorchidism and incomplete testicular descent are congenital abnormalities.
2. Abdominal testes have a high incidence of cancer.
3. Testicular tumors are either germ cell tumors (seminomas [the most common] or nonseminomatous germ cell tumors [embryonal carcinoma, teratoma, choriocarcinoma, or mixed]) or non-germ cell tumors (Leydig and Sertoli cell tumors).
4. Tumors usually manifest as firm, painless testicular masses.
5. Alpha-fetoprotein and beta-human chorionic gonadotropin measurement and ultrasound are used for tumor diagnosis.
6. Orchiectomy, with or without radiation, is standard treatment for testicular tumors.
7. Testicular torsion is caused by abnormally high attachment of the tunica vaginalis around the distal end of the spermatic cord.
8. Testicular torsion is evaluated by Doppler ultrasound because epididymitis can mimic torsion.
9. Testicular torsion requires prompt surgical exploration and bilateral orchiopexy to reverse ischemia from strangulation.

References

Beckman TJ, Mynderse LA. Evaluation and medical management of benign prostatic hyperplasia. *Mayo Clin Proc.* 2005;80(10):1356–1362.

Carver BS, Sheinfeld J. Germ cell tumors of the testis. *Ann Surg Oncol.* 2005;12(11):871–880.

Han M, Partin AW, Pound CR, Epstein JI, Walsh PC. Long-term biochemical disease-free and cancer-specific survival following anatomic radical retropubic prostatectomy. The 15-year Johns Hopkins experience. *Urol Clin North Am.* 2001;28(3):555–565.

BRAIN TUMORS

Because the brain is encased in a nonexpandable bony skull, both benign and malignant brain tumors can cause death if not appropriately diagnosed and treated. Brain tumors cause elevated intracranial pressure (ICP) by occupying space, producing cerebral edema, interfering with the normal flow of cerebrospinal fluid, or impairing venous drainage (Fig. 14-1). Patients present with progressive neurologic deficits due to rising ICP, tumor invasion, or brain compression. Alternatively, they can present with headache or seizures.

PATHOLOGY

Intracranial tumors can be classified as either intracerebral or extracerebral (Table 14-1). Intracerebral tumors include glial cell tumors (astrocytomas, oligodendrogliomas, ependymomas, primitive neuroectodermal tumors), metastatic tumors (lung, breast, melanoma, kidney, colon), pineal gland tumors, and papillomas of the choroid plexus. Extracerebral tumors arise from extracerebral structures and include meningiomas, acoustic neuromas, pituitary adenomas, and craniopharyngiomas.

Glial cell tumors and metastatic tumors are the most common central nervous system (CNS) tumors seen in adults. Children have a higher proportion of posterior fossa tumors.

GLIAL CELL TUMORS

Tumors of glial cells account for approximately 50% of CNS tumors in adults. Different glial cell types (astrocytes, oligodendrocytes, ependymal cells, and neuroglial precursors) give rise to various histologic types of tumors. Although the term *glioma* can be used to describe the above glial tumor types, its common use refers only to astrocytic tumors.

Astrocytic tumors are graded according to histologic evidence of malignancy. Slow-growing astrocytomas are the least malignant and are designated grades I and II. In children, astrocytomas located in the posterior fossa (cerebellum) usually have cystic morphologies (pilocystic astrocytoma). The more aggressive anaplastic astrocytomas are grade III. The most common, as well as the most malignant, astrocytoma is the grade IV glioblastoma multiforme (GBM). GBM tumors often track through the white matter, crossing the midline via the corpus callosum, resulting in the so-called butterfly glioma on computed tomography (CT). Median survival is 1 year.

Oligodendrogliomas are slow-growing calcified tumors, often seen in the frontal lobes. They are most common in adults and are often associated with seizures.

Ependymomas arise from cells that line the ventricular walls and central canal. Clinical signs and symptoms of elevated ICP are the main features of presentation. Ependymomas are mostly seen in children and usually arise in the fourth ventricle.

Infratentorial posterior fossa tumors make up most of the lesions seen in childhood. Cystic cerebellar astrocytomas, ependymomas, and medulloblastomas account for most of these tumors. Highly malignant medulloblastomas are seen in the vermis in children and in the cerebellar hemispheres in young adults.

METASTATIC TUMORS

Approximately 30% of patients with systemic cancer have cerebral metastases, which usually originate in the lung, breast, skin (melanoma), kidney, and colon.

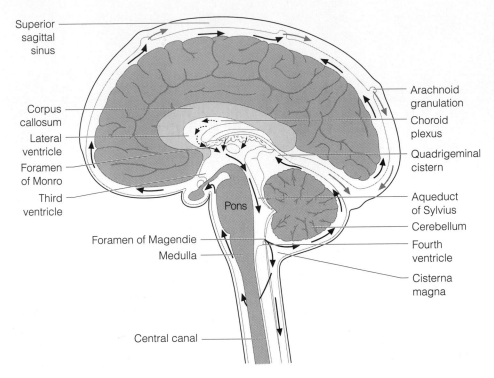

Superior
sagittal
sinus

Corpus
callosum

Lateral
ventricle

Foramen
of Monro

Third
ventricle

Foramen of Magendie

Medulla

Central canal

Pons

Arachnoid
granulation

Choroid
plexus

Quadrigeminal
cistern

Aqueduct
of Sylvius

Cerebellum

Fourth
ventricle

Cisterna
magna

Figure 14-1 • Pathways for the circulation of cerebrospinal fluid.

Most lesions are supratentorial and are located at the cortical white matter junction. Single approachable lesions should be surgically removed, followed by radiation. Stereotactic radiosurgery is used for multiple lesions.

TABLE 14-1 Intracranial Tumors
Intracerebral
Glial cell tumors—astrocytomas, anaplastic astrocytomas, glioblastoma multiforme, oligodendroglioma, ependymoma, primitive neuroectodermal tumors
Metastatic tumors—lung, breast, melanoma, kidney, colon
Pineal gland tumors
Papillomas of the choroid plexus
Extracerebral
Meningiomas
Neuromas, especially acoustic neuromas
Pituitary tumors
Craniopharyngiomas

MENINGIOMAS

Slow-growing meningiomas arise from the meninges lining the brain and spinal cord. Complete tumor removal is curative, and residual disease can be followed or treated with radiosurgery.

History

Patients usually present with neurologic signs and symptoms attributable to cerebral compression from the expanding tumor mass. Seizures are a common presentation. Headache, nausea, vomiting, and mental status changes are the most common generalized symptoms of elevated ICP. Classically, patients complain of diffuse headache that is worse in the morning after a night of recumbency.

Physical Examination

Bilateral papilledema is present at the later stages. Personality changes may be noted early on and may progress to stupor and coma as the ICP increases and brain herniation occurs (Fig. 14-2). Speech deficits and confusion are common with dominant hemisphere

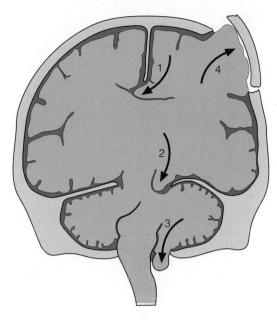

Figure 14-2 • Examples of brain herniation: (1) cingulate gyrus herniation across the falx; (2) temporal uncus herniation across the tentorium; (3) cerebellar tonsil herniation through the foramen magnum; (4) herniation of brain tissue through craniotomy defect.

lesions. Eye deviation can be a sign of frontal lobe involvement. Ataxia is common with cerebellar tumors. Motor or sensory deficits indicate involvement around the central sulcus or deep structures, especially if combined with mental status changes.

Differential Diagnosis

The differential diagnosis for a patient presenting with central neurologic deficits and symptoms includes intracerebral hemorrhage, neurodegenerative diseases, abscess, vascular malformations, meningitis, encephalitis, communicating hydrocephalus, and toxic state.

Diagnostic Evaluation

CT and magnetic resonance imaging (MRI) assist in making the diagnosis and in localization of the tumor. MRI with gadolinium enhancement is useful for visualizing higher-grade gliomas, meningiomas, schwannomas, and pituitary adenomas. T2-weighted MRI is useful for low-grade gliomas.

Treatment

Correct management of brain tumors requires knowledge of the natural history of specific tumor types and the risks associated with surgical removal. When feasible, total tumor removal is the goal; however, subtotal resection may be necessary if vital brain function is threatened by complete tumor extirpation. If subtotal resection is performed, postoperative radiation therapy can prolong life and palliate symptoms. Chemotherapy is also used for specific tumor types.

Metastatic brain tumors are treated with whole-brain irradiation. Occasionally, single lesions amenable to surgery are removed first, followed by whole-brain irradiation.

Perioperative management of increased ICP due to cerebral edema is accomplished by using corticosteroids (dexamethasone [Decadron]). If hydrocephalus is present, shunting of cerebrospinal fluid may be required.

🔑 14-1 KEY POINTS

1. Brain tumors cause elevated intracranial pressure by occupying space, producing cerebral edema, blocking cerebrospinal fluid flow, or impairing cerebral venous drainage, resulting in neurologic deficits.
2. Intracranial tumors are either intracerebral or extracerebral.
3. Glioblastoma multiforme tumors are the most common and most malignant astrocytic tumors. They can track across the corpus callosum and are therefore called butterfly gliomas.
4. Most childhood tumors are located in the posterior fossa and are cystic astrocytomas, ependymomas, and medulloblastomas.

INTRACRANIAL ANEURYSMS

Intracranial aneurysms are saccular, berry-shaped aneurysms, usually found at the arterial branch points within the circle of Willis (Fig. 14-3). Although they rarely rupture, significant morbidity and mortality may result secondary to hemorrhage. Subarachnoid hemorrhage (SAH) develops when intracranial aneurysms rupture and bleed.

HISTORY

Sudden onset of a severe headache, typically described as the "worst headache of my life," usually signals the rupture of an intracranial aneurysm. ICP transiently rises with each cardiac contraction, causing a pulsating

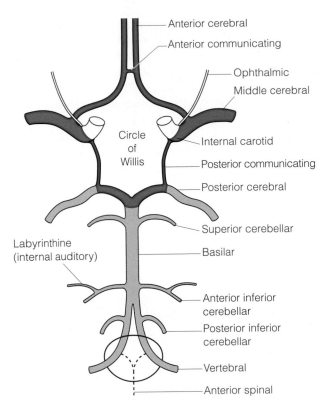

Figure 14-3 • Cerebral arterial circle of Willis.

headache. Progressive neurologic deficits may develop as a result of blood clot mass effect, vasospasm with infarction, or hydrocephalus. Coma and death may occur.

A system for categorizing the severity of hemorrhage has been developed using clinical assessment based on neurologic condition. The five-point Hunt-Hess grading system ranges from grade 1, indicating good neurologic condition, to grade 5, indicating significant neurologic deficits (Table 14-2).

■ **TABLE 14-2** Hunt-Hess Classification of Subarachnoid Hemorrhage	
Grade	**Description**
1	Mild headache and slight nuchal rigidity
2	Cranial nerve palsy, severe headache, nuchal rigidity
3	Mild focal deficit, lethargy or confusion
4	Stupor, hemiparesis, early decerebrate rigidity
5	Deep coma, decerebrate rigidity, moribund appearance

DIAGNOSIS

CT is useful for demonstrating SAH. If CT is negative in a patient with a highly suspicious presentation, a lumbar puncture should be performed. If SAH is present, four-vessel cerebral angiography is performed to define the aneurysm neck and relationship with surrounding vessels (Fig. 14-4).

TREATMENT

Initial medical treatment involves control of hypertension with intravenous medications. Phenytoin is administered for prophylactic treatment of seizures, mannitol can be given to control edema, and nimodipine

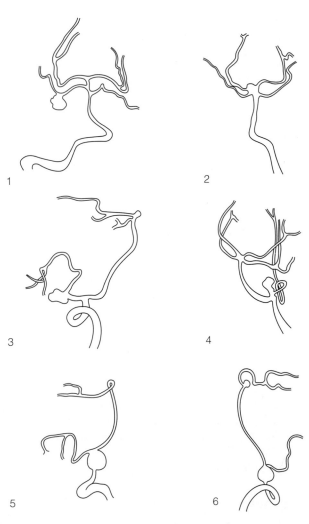

Figure 14-4 • Drawings of six intracranial aneurysms as shown on vertebral angiograms.

is used to reduce the risk of developing delayed neurologic deficits from vasospasm.

Emergency external ventricular drainage may be indicated to lower the ICP. In rare cases with progressive neurologic deterioration, emergency craniotomy and evacuation of a blood clot are required to prevent herniation. The definitive treatment is obliteration by microsurgical clipping or endovascular coiling of the aneurysm.

🔑 14-2 KEY POINTS

1. Intracranial aneurysms are usually found at arterial branch points within the circle of Willis.
2. Rupture causes severe headache and subarachnoid hemorrhage
3. Patients with low-grade presentations should have early aneurysm obliteration to prevent rerupture. Patients with high-grade presentations are stabilized with external ventricular drainage, and the aneurysm is obliterated early or in a delayed fashion, depending on brain swelling. Endovascular treatment is frequently considered for higher-grade patients.

EPIDURAL HEMATOMA

Epidural hematomas are usually seen in patients with head trauma who have sustained a skull fracture across the course of the middle meningeal artery, causing an arterial laceration and an expanding hematoma (Fig. 14-5). The increasing pressure of the arterial-based hematoma strips the dura mater from the inner table of the skull, producing a lens-shaped mass capable of causing brain compression and herniation.

HISTORY

Often, the patient has sustained head trauma with loss of consciousness without a persistent neurologic deficit. After a several-hour "honeymoon" period, the patient experiences a rapidly progressive deterioration in level of consciousness.

PHYSICAL EXAMINATION

Assessing the level of consciousness is the most important aspect in evaluating head injuries. The

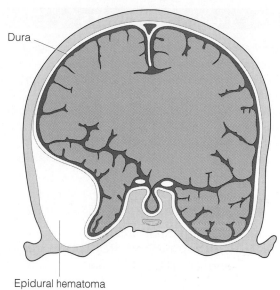

Dura

Epidural hematoma

Figure 14-5 • Epidural hemorrhage.

standard clinical tool for assessment is the Glasgow Coma Scale (GCS), which evaluates eye opening, verbal response, and motor response. Patients with a GCS of 7 or less have severe head injuries, those with scores of 8 to 12 have moderate injuries, and those with scores of more than 12 have mild injuries. Patients with severe injuries (GCS <8) require immediate endotracheal intubation for airway protection and rapid neurosurgical evaluation.

The finding of a unilateral dilated pupil indicates brainstem herniation, whereas bilateral fixed and dilated pupils signal impending respiratory failure and death.

DIAGNOSTIC EVALUATION

CT is crucial to establish a diagnosis and treatment plan.

TREATMENT

For patients presenting with a depressed skull fracture and a neurologic examination indicating a deteriorating level of consciousness, airway control and emergency cranial decompression must be performed. Burr holes are made over the area of hematoma seen on CT, a flap is quickly turned, and the clot is decompressed, with resultant lowering of the ICP. Middle meningeal artery bleeding is controlled, and the dura is fixed to the bone to prevent reaccumulation.

SUBDURAL HEMATOMA

In contrast with epidural hematomas, subdural hematomas are usually low-pressure bleeds secondary to venous hemorrhage (Fig. 14-6). Both spontaneous and traumatic subdural bleeds occur. The source of hemorrhage is from ruptured bridging veins that drain blood from the brain into the superior sagittal sinus.

RISK FACTORS

Elderly patients with evidence of brain atrophy who take anticoagulation medications are at risk for developing spontaneous subdural hematomas.

HISTORY

Headache, drowsiness, and hemiparesis are the usual presenting symptoms. Seizure activity and papilledema are uncommon. Patients with significant neurologic deficits secondary to mass effect may need urgent burr-hole decompression or craniotomy.

SPINAL TUMORS

Tumors are defined by anatomic location as being extradural, intradural, or intramedullary (Fig. 14-7). Extradural tumors are most commonly lesions of metastatic disease from primary cancers of the lung, breast, or prostate. Other common tumors are multiple myeloma of the spine and lymphoma. Back pain or neurologic deficit from cord compression is the usual presenting complaint.

The most common intradural tumors are meningiomas, schwannomas, neurofibromas, and ependymomas. A nerve root tumor may transverse the intervertebral foramen, forming a bilobed lesion called a *dumbbell tumor*. Patients usually present with numbness progressing to weakness.

Intramedullary tumors include astrocytomas, ependymomas, and cavernous malformations. It is important to differentiate cystic tumors from syringomyelia by gadolinium-enhanced MRI, because both may present with sensory loss.

DIFFERENTIAL DIAGNOSIS

The differential diagnosis for patients presenting with signs and symptoms of spinal cord pathology are cervical spondylitic myelopathy, acute cervical disc protrusion, spinal angioma, and acute transverse myelitis.

PHYSICAL EXAMINATION

Patients with tumors of the spine typically present with complaints indicative of progressive spinal cord compression, with evidence of a sensory level.

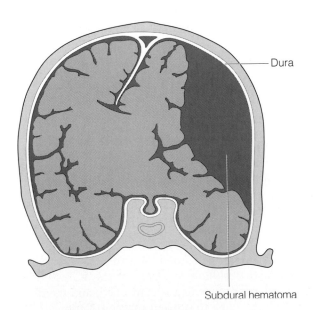

Dura

Subdural hematoma

Figure 14-6 • Subdural hemorrhage.

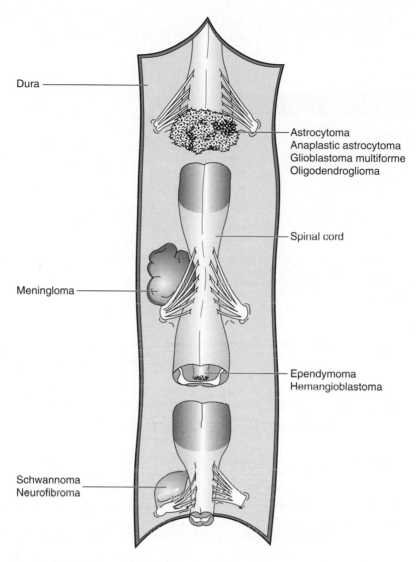

Figure 14-7 • Topographic distribution of the common neoplasms of the spinal meninges, spinal nerve roots, and spinal cord.

DIAGNOSTIC EVALUATION

Plain radiographs may demonstrate bony erosion. MRI is the modality of choice, because it provides detailed anatomic definition. A CT myelogram is done if MRI is unavailable.

TREATMENT

The goal of spinal tumor treatment is to relieve cord compression and to maintain spinal stability. These are interrelated goals, because removing a compressing tumor usually requires surgery on the vertebral column.

The spine consists of two columns: the anterior column (vertebral bodies, discs, and ligaments) and the posterior column (facet joints, neural arch, and ligaments). Damage sustained to one of the columns may result in permanent spinal instability.

For anterior tumors that involve the vertebral body, tumor removal via the anterolateral approach is performed. The vertebral body is resected and the defect repaired with a bone graft and metal plate stabilization.

Posterior tumors can be removed by laminectomy that usually does not cause spinal instability. Metastatic and unresectable disease can be palliated and pain controlled with radiation therapy. Occasionally, anterior and posterior approaches are combined; therefore, appropriate spine stabilization requirements must be anticipated.

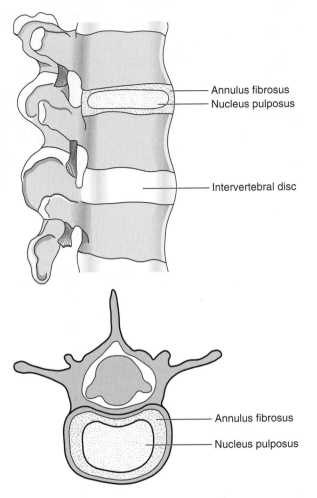

Figure 14-8 • Intervertebral disc: annulus fibrosus and centrally located nucleus pulposus.

🔑 14-5 KEY POINTS

1. Spinal tumors are extradural, intradural, or intramedullary.
2. Most extradural tumors are metastatic lesions.
3. Symptoms of pain, myelopathy, disc protrusion, spinal angioma, and transverse myelitis.
4. Anterior and posterior surgical approaches are used.

SPONDYLOSIS AND DISC HERNIATION

Degenerative changes in the spine are responsible for a large proportion of spine disease. Intervertebral discs consist of two parts: the central nucleus pulposus, which acts as a cushion between vertebrae, and the surrounding dense annulus fibrosus (Fig. 14-8). At birth, the nucleus contains 80% water, but by adulthood, it begins to dehydrate, and disc space narrowing occurs. In the cervical and lumbar spines, disc space narrowing causes abnormal vertebral stresses and movement, which in turn cause osteogenesis, with the formation of osteophytes and bony spurs. These degenerative bone growths can traumatize nerve roots. This degenerative process secondary to abnormal motion in an aging spine is called *spondylosis*.

Structural failure of the intervertebral disc occurs when the nucleus pulposus herniates into the spinal canal or the neural foramina through a defect in the circumferential disc annulus. Lateral disc herniation can cause nerve root compression and radicular symptoms; central disc herniation can cause myelopathy.

These two interrelated degenerative processes are responsible for most spine disease, manifested by nerve root and spinal cord compression. The most mobile segments of the spine (cervical and lumbar) are commonly affected by both processes (Fig. 14-9).

HISTORY

Patients with cervical spondylosis and disc disease are typically older than 50 years and can present with complaints of pain, paresthesia, or weakness. In the case of cervical spondylotic myelopathy secondary to repetitive

spinal cord damage by osteophytes, patients experience progressive numbness, weakness, and paresthesia of the hands and forearms in a glovelike distribution. In contrast, patients with radiculopathy secondary to disc disease complain of pain radiating down the arm in a nerve root distribution, worsening on neck extension.

PHYSICAL EXAMINATION

Limitation of neck motion and straightening of the normal cervical lordosis are common findings. Sensory and motor deficits in a radicular pattern and careful testing for signs of diminished biceps, brachioradialis, and triceps reflexes assist with localization. Hyperreflexia and the presence of the Hoffmann or Babinski reflex help determine the presence of myelopathy and are important signs to elicit.

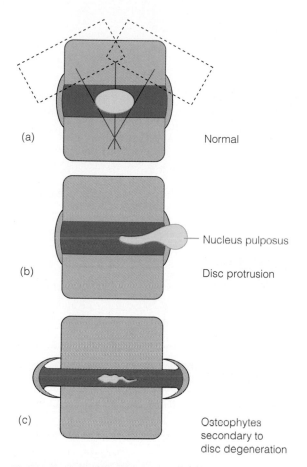

(a) Normal

(b) Nucleus pulposus

Disc protrusion

(c) Osteophytes
secondary to
disc degeneration

Figure 14 9 · Diagram **(a)** shows normal disc space with normal rotatory movement of one vertebra on the adjacent one. Diagram **(b)** shows a disc protrusion, whereas diagram **(c)** shows osteophytes developing secondary to disc degeneration (or disc protrusion). Note the different origin of the disc protrusion and osteophytes.

DIFFERENTIAL DIAGNOSIS

All causes of cervical spinal cord or cervical nerve root compression must be considered. More common causes of cord compression are rheumatoid arthritis and ankylosing spondylitis. For nerve root compression, brachial plexus compression from a first or cervical rib and scalenus anticus syndromes (thoracic outlet syndrome) should be ruled out. Peripheral nerve entrapment (carpal tunnel syndrome, ulnar nerve palsy) and Pancoast tumor of the pulmonary apex should be considered in patients who have arm pain without neck pain.

DIAGNOSTIC EVALUATION

Cervical spine x-rays show straightening of the normal cervical lordosis, disc space narrowing, osteophyte

formation, and spinal canal narrowing. If the axial diameter of the cervical spinal canal is 10 mm or less, risk is high for cervical cord compression.

CT myelography and MRI are used to evaluate the spinal cord and nerve roots and define their relationships to other vertebral structures. Areas of cord and root compression can be identified and intervention planned. MRI is the study of choice for initial evaluation of a herniated cervical disc, whereas CT is preferred when more bony detail is required.

TREATMENT

All patients should initially be managed with medical therapy, except for those with myelopathy or severe radicular weakness. Cervical traction, analgesics, and muscle relaxants are used. For acute cervical radiculopathy due to cervical disc herniation, more than 95% of patients improve without surgery. However, patients with spondylosis and disc prolapse who fail to improve or who exhibit progressive worsening may require surgical treatment.

Because the pathogeny of degenerative osteogenesis is abnormal stress and movement between vertebrae, procedures aimed at stabilizing the spine have shown significant success in obtaining symptomatic relief and promoting osteophyte reabsorption. Anterior cervical fusion produces immobilization by removal of the intervertebral disc, with bone graft replacement and internal fixation. Both cervical spondylosis and cervical disc prolapse can be treated with this procedure.

Decompression laminectomy is usually performed only on patients who have a diffusely narrow spinal canal and who are rapidly worsening due to spondylotic myelopathy. The posterior approach for lateral disc herniations is also used to avoid segmental fusion.

LUMBAR DISC DISEASE

Lumbar disc prolapse is a common disorder. Patients often present with pain radiating down the lower extremity.

Physical Examination

Symptoms of sciatica are caused by disc herniation compression of a nerve root, leading to severe radicular pain. The L4-5 and L5-S1 discs most commonly prolapse, leading to L5 and S1 nerve root symptoms. Paresthesia, numbness, and weakness may be present. Straight leg raise testing can be positive for pain radiating down the affected extremity, with both ipsilateral and contralateral leg raising. Other important signs indicating disc herniation include absence of an ankle or knee reflex, weakness of foot dorsiflexion or plantar flexion, or weakness of knee extension.

Diagnosis

Clinical diagnosis is confirmed by MRI that demonstrates disc protrusion at the suspected level (Fig. 14-10).

Treatment

Most patients improve without surgery; one indication for elective surgery, however, is chronic, disabling, intractable pain. The standard procedure of choice is open laminectomy and discectomy of the appropriate interspace. Urgent surgery is indicated in patients with progressive neurologic deficits (e.g., foot drop) and in those with acute onset of cauda equina syndrome (CES), which is a neurosurgical emergency and occurs as a result of a massive midline disc protrusion that compresses the cauda equina. Typical findings of CES include urinary retention or overflow incontinence, bilateral sciatica, and perineal numbness and tingling (i.e., saddle anesthesia). Urgent bilateral laminectomy decompression with disc removal is required.

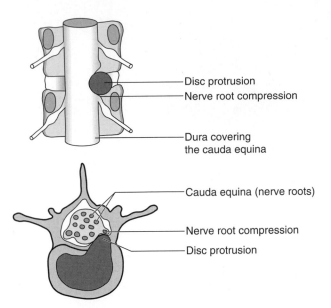

Figure 14-10 • The relations of a lumbar disc prolapse. The protruding disc causes nerve root compression.

🔑 14-6 KEY POINTS

1. Spondylosis and disc herniation can manifest with nerve root or spinal cord compression.
2. Most patients with spondylosis and disc herniation improve without surgery.
3. Cauda equina syndrome presents as urinary retention or overflow incontinence, bilateral sciatica, and perineal numbness secondary to lumbar disc herniation. Urgent decompressive laminectomy is indicated.

References

Bergen MS, Keles GE. Advances in neurosurgical technique in the current management of brain tumors. *Semin Oncol.* 2004;31(5):659–665.

DeAngelis LM. Medical progress: brain tumors. *N Eng J Med.* 2001;344:114–123.

Deyo RA, Weinstein JN. Primary care: low back pain. *N Eng J Med.* 2001;344:363–370.

BASIC SCIENCE

Organ transplantation is one of the great achievements of 20th-century medicine. Fueled by technological advances in immunology and surgical technique, transplantation of the kidney, heart, and liver is now commonplace. Lung, pancreas, and small intestinal transplants are also possible.

The key to successful organ transplantation is the ability to control the immunologic reaction when a donor's tissues are rejected by the recipient's body (Table 15-1). The host's response to the donor's major histocompatibility antigens is the key factor in the success or failure of organ transplantation. Major histocompatibility antigens are coded by a single chromosomal complex called the *major histocompatibility complex* (MHC). In humans, the MHC is named the *HLA antigen* (human leukocyte antigen), which is found on the short arm of chromosome 6. HLA antigens are classified according to their structure and function. Class I antigens are present on virtually all nucleated cells in the human body and act as targets for cytotoxic T cells. Class II antigens are located only on B cells, monocytes, macrophages, and activated T cells and are important in antigen presentation. The rejection reaction of a transplant recipient directed against mismatched donor HLA antigens is a complex event that involves the actions of cytotoxic T cells, activated helper T cells, B lymphocytes, activated macrophages, and antibodies. The reaction is primarily cellular in nature and is T cell–dependent. Class I antigens stimulate cytotoxic T cells, directly causing donor tissue destruction. Class II antigens activate helper T cells, which, along with activated cytotoxic T cells, elaborate interleukin-1 (IL-1) and IL-2. IL-1 and IL-2, in turn, further activate macrophages and antibody-releasing B cells.

Though most rejections are cell-mediated, humoral rejections are also possible. In general, humoral rejections occur early after transplantation because of preformed antibodies against class I antigens in the recipient. These antibodies are commonly acquired via blood transfusions, pregnancy, or prior transplants. When this rejection occurs in the period immediately following the transplant, it is termed *hyperacute rejection*. To avoid this rejection, crossmatching of the recipient's serum against the donor's lymphocytes is necessary to confirm the presence of pre-existing antibodies against donor tissue antigens. Types of rejection are given in Table 15-1.

Immunosuppressive regimens employ a combination of agents among a number of classes. Most patients are on three drug regimens. Currently, the foundation of immunosuppression is a calcineurin inhibitor (either tacrolimus or cyclosporine). This agent binds to immunophilins and inhibits calcineurin activity, which is necessary for the transcription of genes that activate T cells, including IL-2, IL-3, IL-4, and interferon (IFN). Steroids are commonly used in addition, because they alter the transcription and translation of several genes responsible for cytokine synthesis; they inhibit T cell activation by blocking IL-1, IL-2, IL-6, and IFN synthesis; and they have local anti-inflammatory effects. Finally, an antimetabolite, such as mycophenolate mofetil (MMF), is added to the regimen. MMF is rapidly converted to the morpholinoethyl ester of mycophenolic acid (MPA), which inhibits inosine monophosphate dehydrogenases, thus blocking proliferation of T and B lymphocytes and inhibiting antibody formation and the generation of cytotoxic T cells. MPA also downregulates the expression of adhesion molecules on lymphocytes. Other drugs in this category include azathioprine, a purine synthesis inhibitor, and Cytoxan, an alkylating agent.

TABLE 15-1 Classification Criteria for Allograft Rejection Responses

Type	Time Course	Target	Response
Hyperacute	Minutes to hours	Vessels	Humoral
Acute	Early after transplant	Parenchyma/vessels	Cellular/humoral
Chronic	Late after transplant	Parenchyma/vessels	Cellular/humoral

Specific antibodies are now available against T and B cells and are commonly used as induction agents to decrease the risk of acute rejection, as well as to treat rejection. These antibodies include antithymocyte globulin and OKT3, which specifically bind to T cells and tag them for destruction by the reticuloendothelial system. It is unusual for these tremendously potent drugs to fail to stop a rejection.

LIVER TRANSPLANTATION

EPIDEMIOLOGY

There are almost 20,000 patients on the waiting list for liver transplants in the United States, and 5,000 people on the waiting list die each year.

INDICATIONS

Liver transplantation is indicated for life-threatening or debilitating liver failure or early-stage hepatocellular cancer that is not resectable due to tumor location or underlying liver disease. Disease states leading to end-stage liver disease are listed in Table 15-2.

LIVER ALLOCATION

Assignment of livers to patients depends on the Model for End-Stage Liver Disease (MELD), a formula that uses the patient's creatinine, international normalized ratio (INR) of prothrombin time, and bilirubin.

$$MELD = 10(0.957\ln[\text{creatinine mg/dl}] \\ + 0.378\ln[\text{bilirubin mg/dl}] \\ + 1.12\ln[\text{INR}])$$

Values <1.0 are set to 1.0; maximum creatinine that may be used is 4.0, which is also the score for dialysis patients. Ln is the natural logarithm.

This equation produces a number that directly correlates with mortality; livers are offered to the patients with highest mortality. Waiting time is no longer a factor in liver allocation, unless patients have identical MELD scores. This system has been prospectively analyzed and has resulted in fewer deaths on the waiting list. Extra points are offered for certain early-stage tumors in recognition of excellent outcomes with liver transplantation.

TABLE 15-2 Categories of Liver Disease Leading to Transplant

Categories of Disease	Examples
Noncholestatic cirrhosis	Hepatitis B
	Hepatitis C
	Alcoholic cirrhosis
	Autoimmune hepatitis
	Nonalcoholic steatohepatitis
Cholestatic cirrhosis	Primary biliary cirrhosis
	Primary sclerosing cholangitis
	Caroli disease
Metabolic	Wilson disease
	Alpha-1-antitrypsin deficiency
	Tyrosinemia
	Ornithine carbamoyltransferase deficiency
Cancer	Hepatoblastoma
	Hepatoma
Congenital	Biliary atresia
Acute fulminant liver failure	Tylenol overdose
	Halothane hepatitis
	Cryptogenic cirrhosis
Miscellaneous	Budd-Chiari syndrome
	Polycystic liver disease
	Large adenomas

PROGNOSIS

Patient survival after liver transplantation is 93% at 3 months, 88% at 1 year, 80% at 3 years, and 74% at 5 years. Graft survival rates are 88% at 3 months, 81% at 1 year, and 66% at 5 years. Fulminant hepatic failure carries the worst prognosis after transplantation.

After successful liver transplantation, many patients return to a normal life, including work.

THE OPERATION: LIVER TRANSPLANT

Before beginning, it is imperative that adequate blood, platelets, and fresh frozen plasma are available. After the organ is verified to be the correct ABO type, the entire abdomen is prepped, as is the groin in case bypass will be necessary. Intravenous antibiotics are administered, and central monitoring is established. A wide bilateral subcostal incision with midline extension is made. Goals are dissecting the suprahepatic cava, isolating the portal vein in the porta hepatis, and freeing the liver from the diaphragm above the bare area of the liver. The liver can be removed with or without the inferior vena cava. If the liver is removed from the cava, the hepatic veins are clamped and the new liver is sewn so it "hangs down" from the hepatic veins (piggyback technique). In this case, the cava is never divided. If the cava is removed (straight orthotopic), the new liver is sewn to the supra- and infrahepatic portions of the cava. The portal vein is then reconstructed, followed by the hepatic artery and finally the bile duct. Drains are placed, and the abdomen is closed.

KIDNEY TRANSPLANTATION

EPIDEMIOLOGY

There are currently more than 60,000 people in the United States waiting for a kidney transplant, among a group of more than 300,000 patients on dialysis.

INDICATIONS

Kidney transplantation is indicated for end-stage renal disease in patients otherwise healthy enough to tolerate the surgery and subsequent immunosuppression. Common causes are given in Table 15-3.

KIDNEY ALLOCATION

Kidney allocation is based on a formula that incorporates the kidney's degree of match, the waiting time, whether a person has been a kidney donor, the recipient's age, and the recipient's degree of sensitization (Table 15-4).

PROGNOSIS

The half-life of a cadaver kidney, censoring for patient death, is more than 10 years, whereas for a live donor kidney, it is close to 30 years. Transplantation is superior to dialysis for quality of life and survival, even in older people.

■ TABLE 15-3 Disease States Leading to End-Stage Renal Disease
Glomerulonephritis
Chronic pyelonephritis
Hereditary conditions—polycystic kidney disease; nephritis, including Alport syndrome; tuberous sclerosis
Metabolic conditions—diabetes mellitus, hyperoxaluria, cystinosis, Fabry disease, amyloid, gout, porphyria
Obstructive uropathy
Toxic insults
Multisystem disease (lupus, vasculitis, scleroderma)
Hemolytic-uremic syndrome
Tumors
Congenital—hypoplasia, horseshoe
Irreversible ATN
Trauma
Recurrences That Cause Graft Loss
FSGS: 30%
Mesangiocapillary type I glomerulonephritis: 20%
Hemolytic-uremic syndrome: 50%
Oxalosis: 90%
Recurrences That Do Not Result in Graft Loss (generally)
Membranous glomerulonephritis
IgA nephropathy
ATN, acute tubular necrosis; FSGS, Focal segmental glomerulosclerosis; IgA, immunoglobulin A.

TABLE 15-4 Kidney Allocation	
Criteria	**Number of Points**
Each year on the waiting list	1
Very high preformed antibodies	4
<10 years old	4
11–17 years old	3
Previous organ donor	4
No mismatch	7
One mismatch	5
Two mismatches	2

THE OPERATION: KIDNEY TRANSPLANT

Before beginning, it is imperative to verify that the proper kidney has been received and is ABO compatible and crossmatch negative. Placement of the kidney on the right side is usually easier, as the right iliac vein is more accessible than the left for anastomosis. Incising from the pubis to two finger-breadths medial to the anterior-superior iliac spine allows exposure of the anterior rectus sheath and the external oblique. Incision through the muscular and fascial layers permits entry into the retroperitoneal space. Care is taken to preserve the spermatic cord in males.

Dissection of the retroperitoneal space allows the renal vessels to be anastomosed to the external iliac artery and vein. Anastomosis of the ureter directly to the bladder re-establishes drainage.

🔑 15-1 KEY POINTS

1. Control of the host response to donor major histocompatibility antigens is the key to successful organ transplantation.
2. In humans, the major histocompatibility complex is called the *HLA antigen* (human leukocyte antigen).
3. HLA antigens are either class I or class II.
4. Class I antigens are targets for cytotoxic T cells, whereas class II antigens are important in antigen presentation.
5. Tissue rejection is primarily a function of cellular immunity.
6. Hyperacute rejection is a function of humoral responses to HLA antigen or ABO mismatching.
7. Immunosuppressives are used to control or prevent the rejection reaction.
8. Liver transplantation is indicated for end-stage liver disease or unresectable early stage hepatocellular cancer.
9. Liver transplantation is a lifesaving procedure, as most patients will die without a transplant.
10. Kidney transplantation improves quality of life and extends life, as compared with dialysis.

References

Busuttil RW, Klintmalm GB, eds. *Transplantation of the Liver.* 2nd ed. Philadelphia, PA: WB Saunders; 2005.

Danovitch GM, ed. *Handbook of Kidney Transplantation.* 3rd ed. Philadelphia, PA: Lippincott Williams & Wilkins; 2001.

Pancreas

The pancreas is a key regulator of digestion and metabolism through both endocrine and exocrine functions. Disorders of surgical importance include acute pancreatitis, chronic pancreatitis, and pancreatic cancer.

EMBRYOLOGY

Formation of the pancreas begins during the first few weeks of gestation, with the development of the ventral and dorsal pancreatic buds. Clockwise migration of the ventral bud allows fusion with the larger dorsal bud, creating the duct of Wirsung, which is the main pancreatic duct (Fig. 16-1). Failure of this process results in pancreas divisum, wherein the duct of Santorini drains a portion of the exocrine pancreas through a separate minor duodenal papilla (Fig. 16-2). This anatomic variant is associated with pancreatitis. Annular pancreas occurs when the ventral bud fails to rotate, resulting in pancreatic tissue completely or partially encircling the second portion of the duodenum. This situation may result in duodenal obstruction, requiring operation in some cases.

ANATOMY AND PHYSIOLOGY

The pancreas is a retroperitoneal structure located posterior to the stomach and anterior to the inferior vena cava and aorta. This yellowish, multilobed gland is divided into four portions: head, which includes the uncinate process; neck; body; and tail (Fig. 16-3). It lies in a transverse orientation, with the pancreatic head in intimate association with the C loop of the duodenum, the body draped over the spine, and the tail nestled in the splenic hilum.

The arterial blood supply to the pancreatic head is derived from the anterior and posterior pancreaticoduodenal arteries (Fig. 16-4). These arteries arise from the superior pancreaticoduodenal artery, which is a continuation of the gastroduodenal artery, and from the inferior pancreaticoduodenal artery, which arises from the superior mesenteric artery. The body and tail are supplied from branches of the splenic and left gastroepiploic arteries. Venous drainage follows arterial anatomy and enters the portal circulation.

Sympathetic innervation is responsible for transmitting pain of pancreatic origin, whereas efferent postganglionic parasympathetic fibers innervate islet, acini, and ductal systems. In patients with intractable pain from chronic pancreatitis who have failed operative drainage or resection, splanchnicectomy (sympathectomy) can be performed to interrupt sympathetic nerve fibers.

The functional units of the endocrine pancreas are the islets of Langerhans, which are multiple small endocrine glands scattered throughout the pancreas that make up only 1% to 2% of the total pancreatic cell mass. The bulk of the pancreatic parenchyma is exocrine tissue. Four islet cell types have been identified: A cells (alpha), B cells (beta), D cells (delta), and F cells (PP cell).

Alpha cells produce glucagon, which is secreted in response to stimulation by amino acids, cholecystokinin (CCK), gastrin, catecholamines, and sympathetic and parasympathetic nerves. The role of alpha cells is to ensure an ample supply of circulating nutritional fuel during periods of fasting. It promotes hepatic gluconeogenesis and glycogenolysis and inhibits gastrointestinal motility and gastric acid secretion.

The largest percentage of islet volume is occupied by the insulin-producing beta cells. The main function

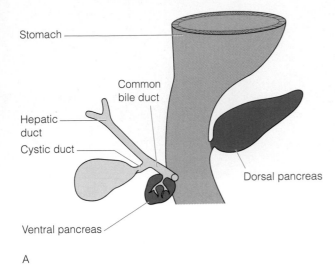

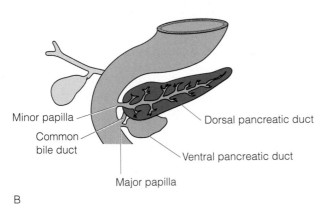

Figure 16-1 • After clockwise rotation in a dorsal direction, the ventral pancreas comes to be adjacent to the dorsal pancreas. The dorsal pancreatic duct enters the duodenum at the minor papilla and the ventral pancreatic duct at the major papilla.

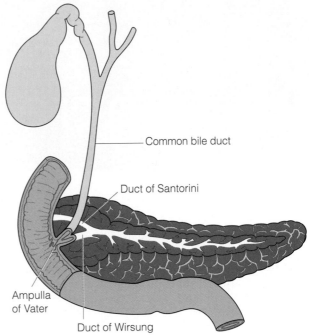

Figure 16-2 • The pancreatic ductal system, including the ducts of Wirsung (major duct) and Santorini (minor duct).

release. Pancreatic somatostatin slows the movement of nutrients from the intestine into the circulation by decreasing pancreatic exocrine function, reducing splanchnic blood flow, decreasing gastrin and gastric acid production, and reducing gastric emptying time. Somatostatin also has paracrine-inhibitory effects on insulin, glucagon, and pancreatic polypeptide (PP) secretion.

F cells secrete PP after ingestion of a mixed meal. The function of PP is unknown; however, it may be important in "priming" hepatocytes for gluconeogenesis. Patients with pancreatic endocrine tumors have been noted to have elevated levels of circulating PP.

The basic functional unit of the exocrine pancreas is the acinus. Acinar cells contain zymogen granules in the apical region of the cytoplasm. Acini are drained by a converging ductal system that terminates

of insulin is to promote the storage of ingested nutrients. Insulin is released into the portal circulation in response to glucose, amino acids, and vagal stimulation. Insulin has both local and distant anabolic and anticatabolic activity. Local paracrine function is the inhibition of glucagon secretion by alpha cells. In the liver, insulin inhibits gluconeogenesis, promotes the synthesis and storage of glycogen, and prevents glycogen breakdown. In adipose tissue, insulin increases glucose uptake by adipocytes, promotes triglyceride storage, and inhibits lipolysis. In muscle, it promotes the synthesis of glycogen and protein.

Somatostatin is secreted by islet delta cells in response to the same stimuli that promote insulin

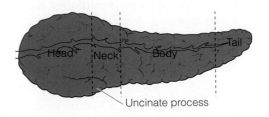

Figure 16-3 • Regional anatomy of the pancreas.

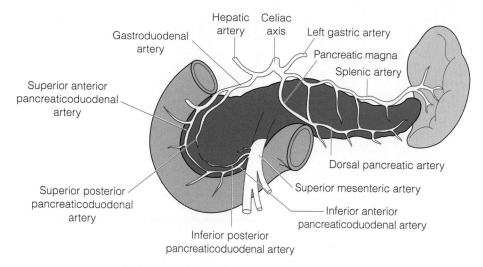

Figure 16-4 • Blood supply of the pancreas

in the main pancreatic excretory duct. The centroacinar cells of individual acini form the origins of the ducts, with intercalated duct cells lining the remainder (Fig. 16-5).

Exocrine pancreatic secretions are products of both ductal and acinar cells. Ductal cells contribute a clear, basic-pH, isotonic solution of water and electrolytes, rich in bicarbonate ions. Secretion of pancreatic fluid is principally controlled by secretin, a hormone produced in the mucosal S cells of the crypts of Lieberkühn in the proximal small bowel. The presence of intraluminal acid and bile stimulates secretin release, which binds pancreatic ductal cell receptors, causing fluid secretion.

Pancreatic digestive enzymes are synthesized by and excreted from acinar cells after stimulation by secretagogues (CCK, acetylcholine). Excreted enzymes include endopeptidases (trypsinogen, chymotrypsinogen, and proelastase) and exopeptidases (procarboxypeptidase A and B). Other enzymes produced are amylase, lipase, and colipase. All peptidases are excreted into the ductal system as inactive precursors. Once in the duodenum, trypsinogen is converted to the active form, trypsin, by interaction with duodenal mucosal enterokinase. Trypsin, in turn, serves to activate the other excreted peptidases (Fig. 16-6). In contrast to the peptidases, the enzymes amylase and lipase are excreted into the ductal system in their active forms.

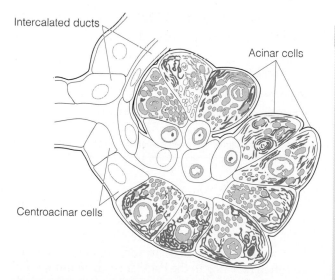

Figure 16-5 • Cellular structure of a pancreatic acinus.

Intercalated ducts

Acinar cells

Centroacinar cells

🔑 16-1 KEY POINTS

1. The pancreas is a retroperitoneal structure consisting of a head, neck, body, and tail.
2. The duct of Wirsung drains the mature pancreas. Occasionally, a duct of Santorini drains through a separate minor papilla.
3. Congenital variants arise from aberrant pancreatic bud migration.
4. The islets of Langerhans of the endocrine pancreas include alpha cells (glucagon), beta cells (insulin), delta cells (somatostatin), and PP cells (pancreatic polypeptide).
5. Trypsinogen is converted to trypsin by duodenal mucosal enterokinase.
6. Trypsin activates the other excreted peptidases.

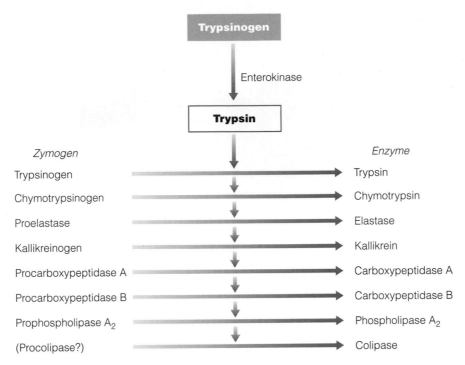

Figure 16-6 • Activation of pancreatic enzymes from the action of trypsin, which is itself activated by the action of enterokinase.

ACUTE PANCREATITIS

PATHOGENESIS

Acute pancreatitis is a disease of glandular enzymatic autodigestion that has varying presentations, ranging from mild parenchymal edema to life-threatening hemorrhagic pancreatitis. Multiple etiologies have been identified, with alcoholism and gallstone disease accounting for 80% to 90% of cases among Western populations. The remaining cases are attributed to hyperlipidemia, hypercalcemia, trauma, infection, ischemia, trauma from endoscopic retrograde cholangiopancreatography (ERCP), and cardiopulmonary bypass (Table 16-1). The exact pathogenesis of acute pancreatitis remains unclear. One possibility is that obstruction of the ampulla of Vater by gallstones, spasm, or edema causes elevated intraductal pressure and bile reflux into the pancreatic duct. Activation and extravasation of intraparenchymal enzymes results in tissue destruction and ischemic necrosis of the pancreas and retroperitoneal tissues.

HISTORY

Because of the different degrees of pancreatic tissue destruction seen in cases of pancreatitis, the presentation

■ TABLE 16-1 Causes of Acute Pancreatitis
Alcohol
Biliary tract disease
Hyperlipidemia
Hypercalcemia
Familial
Trauma—external, operative, ERCP
Ischemic—hypotension, cardiopulmonary bypass
Pancreatic duct obstruction—tumor, pancreas divisum, ampullary stenosis, *Ascaris* infestation
Duodenal obstruction
Infection—mycoplasma, mumps, Coxsackie

ERCP, endoscopic retrograde cholangiopancreatography.

of acute disease is varied, and diagnosis may be difficult. Important past medical history includes information regarding prior episodes of pancreatitis, alcoholism, and biliary colic. Patients present with upper abdominal pain (often radiating to the back), nausea, vomiting, and a low-grade fever. A severe attack of pancreatitis is manifested by hypotension, sepsis, and multiorgan failure.

Patients with an alcoholic etiology usually experience pain 12 to 48 hours after alcohol ingestion.

Patients have upper abdominal tenderness, usually without peritoneal signs. The abdomen may be slightly distended secondary to a paralytic ileus. Low-grade fever and tachycardia are common.

DIFFERENTIAL DIAGNOSIS

Acute pancreatitis is often difficult to differentiate from other causes of upper abdominal pain. The clinical presentation may mimic that of a perforated peptic ulcer or acute biliary tract disease. Other conditions that may have similar presentations are acute intestinal obstruction, acute mesenteric thrombosis, and a leaking abdominal aortic aneurysm.

DIAGNOSTIC EVALUATION

More than 90% of patients who present with acute pancreatitis have an elevated serum amylase. However, amylase levels are relatively nonspecific, because many other intra-abdominal conditions, including intestinal obstruction and perforated peptic ulcer, may cause amylase elevation. If the diagnosis is unclear, a lipase level should also be measured, because it is solely of pancreatic origin.

Leukocytosis >10,000/mL is common, and hemoconcentration with azotemia may also be present because of intravascular depletion secondary to significant third-space fluid sequestration. Hyperglycemia frequently occurs as a result of hypoinsulinemia, and hypocalcemia occurs from calcium deposition in areas of fat necrosis.

Routine chest x-ray may reveal a left pleural effusion, known as a *sympathetic effusion*, secondary to peripancreatic inflammation. Air under the diaphragm indicates perforation of a hollow viscus, such as a perforated peptic ulcer.

The classic radiographic finding on abdominal x-ray is a sentinel loop of dilated mid- to distal duodenum or proximal jejunum located in the left upper quadrant, adjacent to the inflamed pancreas. In cases of gallstone pancreatitis, radiopaque densities (gallstones) may be seen in the right upper quadrant.

Ultrasonography is the preferred modality for imaging the gallbladder and biliary ductal system, because it is more sensitive as compared with computed tomographic (CT) scan. Ultrasound is the study of choice for the detection of cholelithiasis during the workup of gallstone pancreatitis.

CT is the most sensitive radiologic study for confirming the diagnosis of acute pancreatitis. Virtually all patients show evidence of either parenchymal or peripancreatic edema and inflammation. CT is also valuable in defining parenchymal changes associated with pancreatitis, such as pancreatic necrosis and pseudocyst formation. For severe cases, CT scanning with intravenous contrast is important for determining the percentage of pancreatic necrosis, which is a predictor of infectious complications. CT-guided interventional techniques can also be performed to tap peripancreatic fluid collections to rule out infection.

ERCP is useful for imaging the biliary ductal system and can be a diagnostic, as well as a therapeutic, modality. In the case of gallstone pancreatitis, the presence of common bile duct stones (choledocholithiasis) can be confirmed and the stones extracted endoscopically. Magnetic resonance cholangiopancreatography is a newer noninvasive technique that is a diagnostic, but not therapeutic, modality.

DISEASE SEVERITY SCORES

Because the clinical course of pancreatitis can vary from mild inflammation to fatal hemorrhagic disease, prompt identification of patients at risk for development of complications may improve final outcomes. The Ranson criteria are well-known prognostic signs used for predicting the severity of disease based on clinical and laboratory results (Table 16-2). The ability to predict a patient's risk of infectious complications and mortality at the time of admission and during the initial 48 hours allows appropriate therapy to be instituted early in hospitalization. Mortality correlates with the number of criteria present at admission and during the initial 48 hours after admission: 0 to 2

■ TABLE 16-2 Ranson Criteria for Acute Pancreatitis	
At Admission	**During Initial 48 Hours**
Age >55	Hematocrit fall >10%
WBC >16,000	Blood urea nitrogen rise >5
Serum glucose >200	Calcium fall to <8
Serum LDH >350	Arterial PO2 <60
SGOT >250	Base deficit <4
	Fluid sequestration >6 L

LDH, lactic acid dehydrogenase; SGOT, serum glutamic oxaloacetic transaminase.

criteria, 1% mortality; 3 to 4, 16%; 5 to 6, 40%; and 7 to 8, 100%. Since the publication of the Ranson criteria in 1974, newer severity scores have been developed (APACHE II score) to estimate mortality risk in critically ill patients.

TREATMENT

Medical treatment of pancreatitis involves supportive care of the patient and treatment of complications as they arise. No effective agent exists to reverse the inflammatory response initiated by the activated zymogens. With adequate care, however, most cases are self-limited and resolve spontaneously.

Hydration is the most important early intervention in treating acute pancreatitis, because significant third-spacing occurs secondary to parenchymal and retroperitoneal inflammation. Hypovolemia must be avoided because pancreatic ischemia may quickly develop secondary to inadequate splanchnic blood flow.

Traditional treatment calls for putting the pancreas "to rest" by not feeding the patient (NPO). The goal is to decrease pancreatic stimulation, thereby suppressing pancreatic exocrine function. Nasogastric suction can be instituted to treat symptoms of nausea and vomiting.

Antibiotics should be initiated if there is infected pancreatic necrosis, as confirmed by biopsy. In the absence of this, antibiotics are widely used for pancreatitis, but their efficacy is controversial.

If the severity of disease necessitates a prolonged period of remaining NPO, an alternative method of administering nutrition must be instituted. Intravenous nutrition (total parenteral nutrition/hyperalimentation) is commonly initiated. Once pancreatic inflammation resolves, gradual advancement of oral intake proceeds, beginning with low-fat, high-carbohydrate liquids to avoid pancreatic stimulation.

Oxygen therapy may be necessary for treatment of hypoxia, which often occurs secondary to pulmonary changes thought to be due to circulating mediators. Evidence of atelectasis, pleural effusion, pulmonary edema, and adult respiratory distress syndrome may be seen on chest radiograph.

Surgical treatment of acute pancreatitis is directed at complications that develop secondary to the underlying disease process. During the early phase of pancreatitis, areas of necrosis may form because of tissue ischemia from enzyme activation, inflammation, and edema. Necrotic areas eventually liquefy and may become infected if they are unable to reabsorb and heal. CT scanning with intravenous contrast is the key test for defining the extent of pancreatic necrosis. Nonenhancement of 50% or more of the pancreas on CT scan is a strong predictor for the development of infectious complications. Infected collections require surgical debridement and drainage to avoid fatal septic complications.

Peripancreatic collections that persist after the inflammatory phase has subsided may develop a thickened wall, or "rind." Such collections are called *pancreatic pseudocysts*. To alleviate symptoms or prevent major complications, surgical drainage is usually required for cysts >6 cm in diameter that have persisted for more than 6 weeks. Standard therapy is internal drainage into the stomach, duodenum, or small intestine.

During the later stage of disease, abscess formation may occur. The pathogenesis is a progression: An ischemic parenchyma progresses to necrosis and is seeded by bacteria, with eventual abscess formation. Most bacteria are of enteric origin, and standard antibiotic therapy is insufficient treatment. Proper treatment requires adherence to the surgical adage: "All pus must be drained for healing to occur." If surgical drainage and debridement are not performed, the mortality nears 100%. Percutaneous drainage is usually inadequate, because only the fluid component is removed and the necrotic infected tissue remains.

Hemorrhage secondary to erosion of blood vessels by activated proteases can be a life-threatening complication. Often it is the main hepatic, gastroduodenal, or splenic artery that bleeds. If control is not achieved angiographically, surgical exploration is required.

🔖 16-2 KEY POINTS

1. Acute pancreatitis is mostly caused by alcohol ingestion and gallstone disease in Western populations.
2. Pancreatitis results from glandular autodigestion caused by intraparenchymal enzyme activation.
3. Ranson criteria are used to predict the severity of the disease and to estimate mortality.
4. Pancreatitis is usually self-limiting and resolves with supportive care.
5. Complications such as chronic pseudocyst, abscess, necrosis, or hemorrhage are treated surgically.

CHRONIC PANCREATITIS

Of patients with acute pancreatitis, a very small number progress to chronic pancreatitis. The chronic form of disease is characterized by persistent inflammation that causes destructive fibrosis of the gland. The clinical picture is of recurring or persistent upper abdominal pain with evidence of malabsorption, steatorrhea, and diabetes.

PATHOGENESIS

Chronic pancreatitis can be categorized into two forms: calcific pancreatitis, usually associated with persistent alcohol abuse, and obstructive pancreatitis, secondary to pancreatic duct obstruction. Alcohol-induced calcific pancreatitis is the most common form of disease in Western populations. Proposed mechanisms of disease include ductal plugging and occlusion by protein and mineral precipitates. The resulting inflammation and patchy fibrosis subsequently lead to parenchymal destruction and eventual atrophy of the gland. Obstructive chronic pancreatitis is due to ductal blockage secondary to scarring from acute pancreatitis or trauma, papillary stenosis, pseudocyst, or tumor. This blockage results in upstream duct dilatation and inflammation.

HISTORY

Abdominal pain is the principal presenting complaint and the most frequent indication for surgery. The pain is upper abdominal, is either intermittent or persistent, and frequently radiates to the back. Patients are often addicted to narcotic pain relievers. Other symptoms result from exocrine insufficiency (malabsorption) and endocrine insufficiency (diabetes mellitus).

DIAGNOSTIC EVALUATION

Given the functional reserve of the pancreas, the diagnosis of chronic pancreatitis is best made using imaging techniques that detect pancreatic morphologic changes rather than tests of glandular function. Exocrine function may be evaluated by the secretin-cholecystokinin test, which is now rarely used.

The radiologic signs of chronic pancreatitis include a heterogeneously inflamed or atrophied gland, a dilated and strictured pancreatic duct, and the presence of calculi. Ultrasonography and CT are useful initial imaging procedures; however, ERCP is the most accurate means of diagnosing chronic pancreatitis, because it clearly defines the pathologic changes of the pancreatic ductal system and the biliary tree.

TREATMENT

Effective treatment of chronic abdominal pain is often the focus of care for patients with chronic pancreatitis. Opiates are very useful for controlling visceral pain; however, many patients become opiate-dependent over the long term. Alcohol nerve blocks of the celiac plexus have only moderate success.

Pancreatic exocrine insufficiency is treated with oral pancreatic enzymes, and insulin is used to treat diabetes mellitus. Ethanol intake by the patient must cease.

Surgical intervention is undertaken only if medical therapy has proved unsuccessful in relieving chronic intractable pain. Functional drainage of the pancreatic duct and the resection of diseased tissue are the goals of any procedure. Based on ERCP and CT findings, the correct operation can be planned.

For patients with a "chain of lakes"–appearing pancreatic duct, caused by sequential ductal scarring and dilatation, a longitudinal pancreaticojejunostomy (Puestow procedure) is indicated to achieve adequate drainage. A Roux-en-Y segment of proximal jejunum is anastomosed side-to-side with the opened pancreatic duct, facilitating drainage (Fig. 16-7). Distal pancreatic duct obstruction causing localized distal parenchymal disease is best treated by performing a distal pancreatectomy.

✎ 16-3 KEY POINTS

1. Alcohol use is the most common cause of chronic pancreatitis in the West.
2. Exocrine insufficiency (malabsorption) and endocrine insufficiency (diabetes mellitus) may occur.
3. Surgical treatment includes drainage procedures (longitudinal pancreaticojejunostomy [Puestow procedure]) or pancreatic resection (distal pancreatectomy).

PANCREATIC CANCER

EPIDEMIOLOGY

Pancreatic adenocarcinoma is a leading cause of cancer death, trailing other cancers such as lung and colon. Men are affected more than women, by a 2:1 ratio.

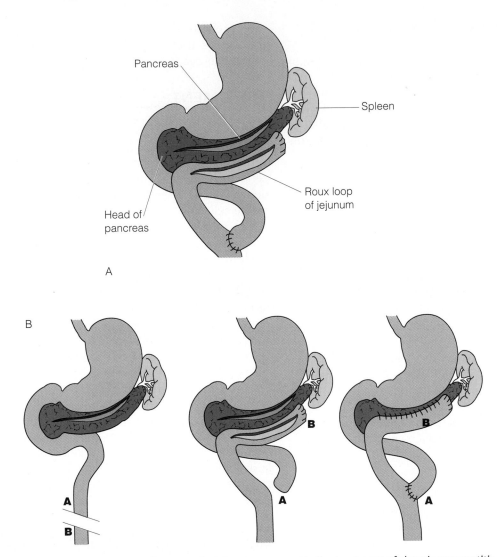

Pancreas

Spleen

Roux loop
of jejunum

Head of
pancreas

A

B

Figure 16-7 • Longitudinal pancreaticojejunostomy used in the treatment of chronic pancreatitis.

Risk factors for development of pancreatic cancer are increasing age and cigarette smoking. The peak incidence is in the fifth and sixth decades. Ductal adenocarcinoma accounts for 80% of the cancer types and is usually found in the head of the gland. Local spread to contiguous structures occurs early, and metastases to regional lymph nodes and liver follow.

HISTORY

The signs and symptoms of carcinoma of the head of the pancreas are intrinsically related to the regional anatomy of the gland. Patients classically complain of obstructive

jaundice, weight loss, and constant deep abdominal pain due to peripancreatic tumor infiltration. Patients may present with jaundice and a palpable nontender gallbladder, indicating tumor obstruction of the distal common bile duct (Courvoisier sign). Pruritus often accompanies the development of jaundice.

DIFFERENTIAL DIAGNOSIS

The differential diagnosis of malignant obstructive jaundice includes carcinomas of the ampulla of Vater, pancreatic head, distal common bile duct, or duodenum.

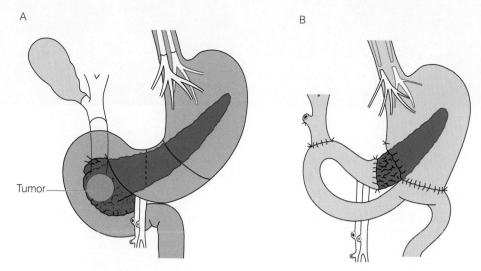

Figure 16-8 • Pancreaticoduodenectomy (Whipple procedure). Preoperative anatomic relationships (A) and postoperative reconstruction (B).

DIAGNOSTIC EVALUATION

The most common laboratory abnormalities are elevated alkaline phosphatase and direct bilirubin levels, indicating obstructive jaundice. The average bilirubin level in neoplastic obstruction is typically higher than that seen in bile duct obstruction from gallstone disease.

CT and ERCP are the modalities of choice for evaluating pancreatic cancer. CT reveals the location of the mass, the extent of tumor invasion or metastasis, and the degree of ductal dilatation. ERCP defines the ductal anatomy and the extent of ductal obstruction and provides biopsy specimens for tissue diagnosis. Drainage stents can be placed into the common bile duct during ERCP for biliary tree decompression. Imaging information suggesting unresectability includes local tumor extension, contiguous organ invasion, superior mesenteric vein or portal vein invasion, ascites, and distant metastases.

TREATMENT

The operation for resectable tumors in the head of the pancreas is pancreaticoduodenectomy (Whipple procedure; Fig. 16-8). This major operation entails the en bloc resection of the antrum, duodenum, proximal jejunum, head of pancreas, gallbladder, and distal common bile duct.

PROGNOSIS

Long-term survival for pancreatic cancer remains dismal, and most patients die within 1 year of diagnosis. The 5-year survival rate for all patients with tumors of the head of the pancreas is approximately 3%. For individuals with tumors amenable to Whipple resection, the 5-year survival rate is only 10% to 20%. Tumors of the body and tail are invariably fatal, because diagnosis is usually made at a more advanced stage due to the lack of early obstructive findings.

🔑 16-4 KEY POINTS

1. In pancreatic cancer, obstructive jaundice, weight loss, and abdominal pain are common findings.
2. The Courvoisier sign is jaundice and a nontender palpable gallbladder, indicating tumor obstruction of the distal common bile duct.
3. Presenting bilirubin levels are typically much higher in malignant biliary obstruction than in common bile duct obstruction from gallstone disease.
4. Computed tomography and endoscopic retrograde cholangiopancreatography are used to determine tumor resectability.
5. Resectable tumors of the head of the pancreas are removed by pancreaticoduodenectomy (Whipple procedure). Prognosis is generally poor.

References

Delbeke D, Pinson CW. Pancreatic tumors: role of imaging in the diagnosis, staging, and treatment. *J Hepatobiliary Pancreatic Surg.* 2004;11(1):4–10.

DiMagno MJ, DiMagno EP. Chronic pancreatitis. *Curr Opin Gastroenterol.* 2005;21(5):544–554.

Pandol SJ. Acute pancreatitis. *Curr Opin Gastroenterol.* 2005;21(5):538–543.

Parathyroid Gland

The surgical treatment of parathyroid disease relates mainly to hyperparathyroidism. Primary hyperparathyroidism results from autonomous parathyroid hormone (PTH) secretion, secondary to glandular hyperplasia; parathyroid adenomas; or, rarely, parathyroid carcinoma. Clinical manifestations of disease are caused by persistent hypercalcemia. Fortunately, the surgical removal of hyperfunctioning glands affords a >90% cure rate.

ANATOMY

Parathyroid glands are small, yellowish-brown ovals, measuring approximately 2 mm × 3 mm × 5 mm. Normal individuals possess four parathyroid glands, although additional glands are possible. Embryonically, the upper paired glands arise from the fourth branchial pouch and are located behind the thyroid gland, in close association with the inferior thyroid artery (Figs. 17-1 and 17-2). The lower two glands, as well as the thymus, arise from the third branchial pouch and are usually located within 2 cm of the lower thyroid pole (Fig. 17-3). The arterial supply to all four glands is from the inferior thyroid artery.

Aberrant migration may produce ectopic parathyroid glands. Based on their embryologic development, aberrant upper glands are usually intrathyroid or posterior mediastinal, whereas aberrant lower glands are usually intrathymic or anterior mediastinal (Fig. 17-4).

PATHOGENESIS

Several forms of hyperparathyroidism exist. Primary hyperparathyroidism results from excess PTH, which causes mobilization of calcium deposits from bone, inhibition of renal phosphate reabsorption, and stimulation of renal tubular absorption of calcium. The result is hypercalcemia and hypophosphatemia. Overall, both total body calcium and phosphate wasting occur, leading to osteoporosis and bony mineral loss. Such metabolic imbalance leads to the development of associated conditions, such as pancreatitis, nephrolithiasis, nephrocalcinosis, gout, pseudogout, hypertension, and peptic ulcer's disease.

Secondary hyperparathyroidism is usually seen in patients with renal's disease, in which hyperphosphatemia causes depression of serum ionized calcium levels. Hypocalcemia then serves to stimulate excess PTH production by glands that typically have become hyperplastic because of the persistent hypocalcemic stimulus.

Tertiary hyperparathyroidism results from long-standing secondary hyperparathyroidism, as persistent hypocalcemia causes the development of autonomous hyperplastic gland function. As in secondary hyperparathyroidism, tertiary disease is seen in dialysis-dependent patients with end-stage renal's disease.

Pseudohyperparathyroidism results in biochemical derangement similar to that seen in primary hyperparathyroidism. Oat cell and squamous cell cancers of the lung, head and neck, kidney, and ovary produce PTH-like proteins that produce a similar picture of hypercalcemia.

EPIDEMIOLOGY

Hyperparathyroidism is the most common cause of hypercalcemia and has an incidence of 0.1% to 0.3% of the population (Table 17-1). The incidence of disease increases with age, and presentations before puberty are uncommon. Women are affected twice as often as men. Approximately 90% of cases are sporadic and are due

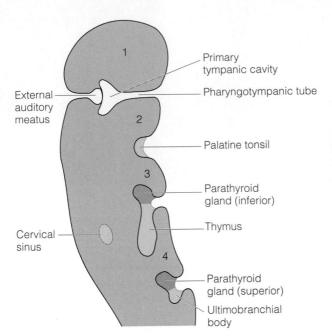

Figure 17-1 • The pharyngeal pouches. The inferior parathyroid arises from the third pouch and the superior arises from the fourth.

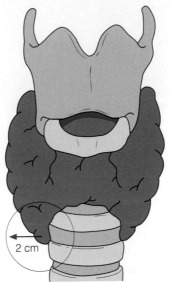

Figure 17-3 • Normal siting of the lower parathyroid glands.

to a single hyperfunctioning adenoma. The remainder are of genetic origin, as hyperparathyroidism is a component of multiple endocrine neoplastic (MEN) disease. Patients with MEN type I (Wermer syndrome) have involvement of the three *p*'s: parathyroid, pituitary, and pancreas. MEN type IIa (Sipple disease) includes hyperparathyroidism, pheochromocytoma, and medullary cancer of the thyroid. Patients with

MEN I or II have diffuse four-gland hyperplasia and require bilateral neck exploration for removal of all affected glands.

RISK FACTORS

Childhood radiation therapy to the head and neck has been proposed as a risk factor for developing hyperparathyroidism. A family history of MEN is also important.

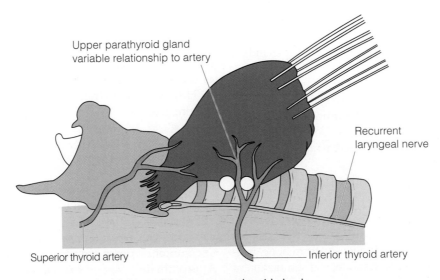

Figure 17-2 • Normal siting of the upper parathyroid glands.

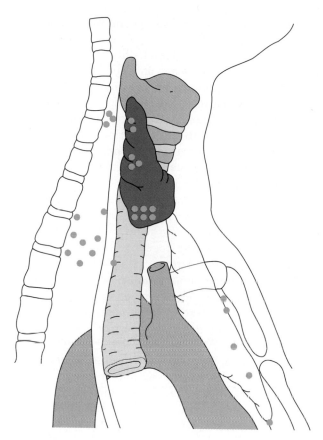

Figure 17-4 • Ectopic parathyroid gland locations, secondary to aberrant migration, found on reoperation for persistent hyperparathyroidism.

■ **TABLE 17-1** Diseases and Factors Causing Hypercalcemia
Hyperparathyroidism
Malignancy
Hyperthyroidism
Multiple myeloma
Sarcoid and other granulomatous diseases
Milk-alkali syndrome
Vitamin D intoxication
Vitamin A intoxication
Paget disease
Immobilization
Thiazide diuretics
Addisonian crisis
Familial hypocalciuric hypercalcemia

HISTORY

Historically, patients with primary hyperparathyroidism presented with advanced end-stage renal disease due to staghorn calculi and obstructive uropathy. Pathologic fractures due to bone reabsorption were typical. Today patients are generally asymptomatic on presentation because diagnosis is usually now made after hypercalcemia is discovered on routine screening. The symptoms of hyperparathyroidism are easily remembered by the time-honored rhyme, "Bones, stones, abdominal groans, psychic moans, and fatigue overtones":

- Bones—Aches and arthralgias result from fractures and structural changes in bony architecture. Pseudogout (chondrocalcinosis) causes severe joint pain when articular cartilage becomes calcified.

- Stones—Renal calculi from hypercalcemia can produce symptoms of renal colic. Calculi can also cause obstructive uropathy, with resulting urinary tract infections and renal failure. Less common is the calcification of the renal parenchyma itself (nephrocalcinosis).
- Abdominal groans—Several abdominal conditions can arise from hypercalcemia. The filtration of high serum calcium loads can cause dehydration and subsequent constipation. Pancreatitis can develop secondary to hypercalcemia. Hypercalcemia is also thought to stimulate gastrin production, which leads to elevated gastric acid secretion. Peptic ulcer disease may also be exacerbated.
- Psychic moans—Hypercalcemia causes anorexia and associated nausea and vomiting. As with constipation, high mineral levels in the kidney cause polyuria, which leads to thirst and polydipsia. Behavioral changes, such as mood swings, organic psychosis, and dementia, can be seen.
- Fatigue overtones—Hypercalcemia can produce a sense of lassitude and muscular fatigability.

PHYSICAL EXAMINATION

Physical examination is generally unremarkable. Occasionally, a neck mass may be palpable. Rarely, localized aggregates of osteoclasts (osteoclastomas, or "brown tumors") can cause focal bone swelling.

DIFFERENTIAL DIAGNOSIS

The differential diagnosis of persistent hypercalcemia includes those diseases and factors listed in Table 17-1. The most common overall cause of hypercalcemia is osseous metastatic disease.

DIAGNOSTIC EVALUATION

The most important finding is persistent hypercalcemia, followed by elevated serum PTH levels. Elevated alkaline phosphatase levels indicate bony disease. Renal function is assessed by creatinine measurement.

Bone films may show evidence of subperiosteal reabsorption of the phalanges, osteopenia, osteoclastomas, and metastatic calcifications. Bone densitometry quantifies osteopenia. Abdominal films may reveal renal calculi or nephrocalcinosis.

TREATMENT

Primary hyperparathyroidism is a surgical disease, and operation is required to remove hyperfunctioning glands. Patients may present in hypercalcemic crisis (coma, delirium, anorexia, vomiting, and abdominal pain), for which vigorous intravenous hydration and forced calciuresis with furosemide are the initial therapy. Once the patient's condition is stabilized and the diagnosis of hyperparathyroidism is confirmed, a surgeon may perform preoperative localization of the parathyroid tumor. The preferred modality is technetium (Tc)-sestamibi scanning, but ultrasonography, CT, or thallium-Tc scanning can also be used. To maximize the success of surgery, preoperative Tc-sestamibi scanning and intraoperative rapid PTH immunoassay are recommended. Once the tumor is removed, PTH levels should decrease to <25% of the baseline value.

The combined use of preoperative Tc-sestamibi scanning and intraoperative rapid PTH assay reportedly results in higher operative success rates and more efficient care. Precise preoperative localization and confirmation of diminished PTH levels after excision decrease operating time, length of stay, and laboratory costs.

The surgical approach for parathyroid procedures is identical to that used for thyroid disease. Through a curvilinear necklace incision, most tumors are usually found attached to the posterior capsule of the thyroid, overlying the recurrent laryngeal nerve and in close proximity to the inferior thyroid artery. All four glands should be identified, because multiple adenomas do occur. In parathyroid hyperplasia, all glands are diseased, which necessitates their surgical removal, except for a single gland, which is subtotally excised. The remaining focus of hyperplastic cells functions to prevent permanent hypocalcemia.

Secondary hyperparathyroidism of renal disease, resulting from low levels of ionized calcium, is treated medically, whereas tertiary hyperparathyroidism, due to autonomous parathyroid hyperplasia, occasionally requires surgical intervention.

After surgery, hypocalcemia occurs secondary to reduced PTH levels and osseous remineralization, known as the "hungry bones" phenomenon. Symptoms of hypocalcemia include periorbital numbness, paresthesia, carpopedal spasm, and seizures. The Chvostek sign can be elicited by gently tapping the facial nerve, causing facial muscle spasm. For mild symptoms of hypocalcemia, treatment consists of oral calcium supplementation and a high-calcium diet. Spasm and seizure activity require immediate treatment with intravenous calcium gluconate or calcium chloride.

Recurrent hyperparathyroidism after the removal of a single adenoma occurs in 5% of cases. Definitive localization should be performed with Tc-sestamibi scanning or other modalities. If localized to the mediastinum, re-exploration is indicated, and sternal split may be necessary. Confirmation of extirpation is by rapid PTH assay.

🔨 17-1 KEY POINTS

1. Hyperparathyroidism is the most common cause of surgically correctable hypercalcemia.
2. Primary hyperparathyroidism results from autonomous parathyroid hormone (PTH) secretion by adenomas, hyperplasia, or carcinoma. A single hyperfunctioning adenoma accounts for approximately 90% of cases.
3. The paired upper glands arise from the fourth branchial pouch, and the lower glands and thymus arise from the third branchial pouch. Aberrant migration produces ectopic parathyroid glands.
4. Excess PTH causes bony calcium mobilization, stimulation of renal calcium reabsorption, and inhibition of renal phosphate absorption. Hypercalcemia and hypophosphatemia occur.
5. Primary hyperparathyroidism is associated with pancreatitis, nephrolithiasis, nephrocalcinosis, gout, pseudogout, hypertension, and peptic ulcer disease.
6. Secondary and tertiary hyperparathyroidism occur in patients with renal disease.
7. Pseudohyperparathyroidism occurs in oat cell and squamous carcinomas that produce PTH-like proteins.
8. Hyperparathyroidism occurs in multiple endocrine neoplastic I and IIa.
9. Symptoms of hyperparathyroidism can be remembered by the rhyme "bones, stones, abdominal groans, psychic moans, and fatigue overtones."
10. Postoperative hypocalcemia ("hungry bones" phenomenon) involves periorbital numbness, paresthesia, carpopedal spasm, seizures, and a positive Chvostek sign.

References

Cailing T, Udelsman R. Parathyroid surgery in familial hyperparathyroid's disorders. *J Intern Med.* 2005;257(1):27–37.

Gutierrez C, Snively CS. Chronic kidney disease: prevention and treatment of common problems. *Am Fam Physician.* 2004;70(10):1921–1928.

Marx SJ. Hyperparathyroid and hypoparathyroid disorders. *N Eng J Med.* 2000;343:1863–1875.

BASAL CELL CARCINOMA

Basal cell carcinoma (BCC) is the most common form of skin cancer in Caucasians. It is rare in Asians and exceedingly rare in darkly pigmented individuals. The predominant etiology is excess exposure to ultraviolet B (UVB) radiation. Accordingly, BCC is a disease of adults, and tumors arise from sun-exposed skin, namely the head and neck. The cellular origin of BCC has traditionally been thought to be the basal cell of the epidermis. More recently, an alternative theory posits that the originating cell type is a pluripotent epithelial cell. BCC is categorized into three types: noduloulcerative, superficial, and sclerosing.

NODULOULCERATIVE BASAL CELL CARCINOMA

Lesions have a pearly, dome-shaped, nodular appearance, with associated telangiectasia and an ulcerated center (Fig. 18-1). Telangiectasia is secondary to tumor-induced angiogenesis, and ulceration results from outgrowth of the local blood supply. Noduloulcerative lesions are the most common type of BCC.

Tumors <1 cm in diameter are rarely invasive and can be treated with cautery and curettage or cryosurgery. Tumors >1 cm are treated with surgical excision. High-risk sites of tumor growth are areas with underlying bone and cartilage (i.e., nose, ear), because the growing tumor tends to track along these structures. Such tumors have a high recurrence rate. Therefore, high-risk tumors and recurrent tumors should be treated with Moh's micrographic surgery to ensure complete excision.

SUPERFICIAL BASAL CELL CARCINOMA

The second most common BCC is the superficial type. Lesions usually appear on the trunk and proximal extremities and clinically resemble thin, scaly, pink plaques with irregular margins (Fig. 18-2). These horizontally expanding tumors are often dismissed as dermatitis; subsequently, tumors reach diameters of several centimeters by the time of diagnosis. By this late stage, ulceration and deep dermal invasion are present. Standard treatment has been wide-margin excision, with skin grafting if necessary. However, this approach may be unacceptably morbid, leaving a large skin defect. Recently, topical chemotherapy with 5-fluorouracil, cryosurgery, and cautery/curettage has shown cure rates similar to those of traditional wide excision.

SCLEROSING BASAL CELL CARCINOMA

Sclerosing BCC is the least common type. The anatomic distribution is similar to that of the noduloulcerative type, but histologically, the lesions appear as narrow cords of tumor cells encased in a proliferation of connective tissue. Macroscopically, lesions are smooth, atrophic, and indurated and easily mimic scar tissue. This deceptive appearance is unfortunate, because sclerosing tumors are more aggressive than other basal cell tumor types. The growth pattern follows tissue planes and neurovascular bundles, resulting in deep soft tissue invasion. Moh's micrographic surgery is the preferred management technique.

MELANOMA

Melanoma is the most frequent cause of death of all skin cancer types. It results from malignant transformation of the normal melanocyte, usually located in the basal layer of the epidermis. Many melanomas are curable by surgical excision.

PATHOGENESIS

Ultraviolet (UV) light is suspected to play a role in the development of all types of skin cancer, including melanoma. Although the precise etiologic role of UV light in the malignant transformation of skin cells remains unresolved, both ultraviolet A (UVA) and UVB are thought to have carcinogenic potential. UVA penetrates deep into the dermis, damaging connective tissue and intrinsic skin elasticity. Excessive UVB exposure results in sunburn.

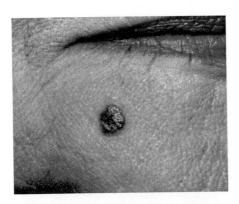

Figure 18-1 • Pigmented basal cell carcinoma. Note the pearly, waxy surface.
From Goodheart HP. *Goodheart's Photoguide of Common Skin Disorders.* 2nd ed. Philadelphia, PA: Lippincott Williams & Wilkins; 2003.

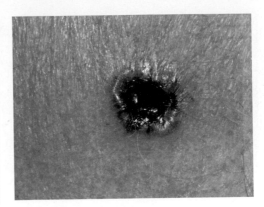

Figure 18-2 • Nodular basal cell carcinoma. Note the rolled borders with telangiectasia.
From Goodheart HP. *Goodheart's Photoguide of Common Skin Disorders.* 2nd ed. Philadelphia, PA: Lippincott Williams & Wilkins; 2003.

EPIDEMIOLOGY

Melanoma accounts for 5% of all skin malignancies and 3% of all cancers. The diagnosis of melanoma carries a 50% mortality in the United States, and the incidence has dramatically increased during the past 10 to 15 years. Most lesions arise from pre-existing moles. A mole that shows rapid growth or heterogeneous pigmentation should be evaluated and possibly biopsied to rule out melanoma. Fair-skinned individuals have a higher incidence of melanoma than does the general population. The five signs of melanoma can be remembered as the ABCDE's: *a*symmetric shape, irregular *b*order, mottled *c*olor, large *d*iameter, and progressive *e*nlargement.

RISK FACTORS

Risk factors include the following: a mole that shows persistent changes in shape, size, or color; persons having more than 100 nevi; atypical nevi (5% of population); personal history or family history of melanoma; excess sun exposure (especially in childhood); fair complexion; and tendency to freckle and sunburn.

MELANOMA TYPES

Superficial spreading melanoma can occur anywhere, on both sun-exposed and nonexposed areas. The average age of diagnosis is 40 to 50 years. Lesions are commonly on the upper back and lower legs. Lesions show heterogeneous pigmentation with irregular margins. The growth phase is radial with horizontal spread (Fig. 18-3).

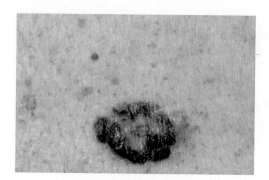

Figure 18-3 • Superficial spreading melanoma. Note the central area (whitish gray) of regression.
From Goodheart HP. *Goodheart's Photoguide of Common Skin Disorders.* 2nd ed. Philadelphia, PA: Lippincott Williams & Wilkins; 2003.

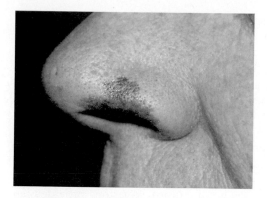

Figure 18-4 • Lentigo maligna melanoma. Biopsy of this lesion demonstrated invasion into the dermis.
From Goodheart HP. *Goodheart's Photoguide of Common Skin Disorders.* 2nd ed. Philadelphia, PA: Lippincott Williams & Wilkins; 2003.

Lentigo maligna melanoma is usually seen in older individuals, with the average age of diagnosis being 70 years. Lesions appear on sun-exposed surfaces, particularly the malar region of the cheek and temple. Lesions exhibit horizontal spread (Fig. 18-4).

Acral lentiginous melanoma has an unusual distribution in that lesions appear on palms, soles, nail beds, or mucous membranes. The most common mucous membrane site is the vulva. Other sites include the anus, nasopharynx, sinuses, and oral cavity. The average age of diagnosis is 60 years. Spread is in a horizontal pattern.

Nodular melanoma can occur at any site and has a very early malignant potential secondary to a predominantly vertical growth phase. In contrast, the three other melanoma types exhibit radial growth phases with horizontal spread. Nodular lesions have well-circumscribed borders and uniform black or brown coloring.

PROGNOSIS

As with other cancers, the extent of spread is an important prognostic factor. Stage I is local disease <1.5 mm. Stage II is local disease >1.5 mm. Stage III is regional disease. Stage IV is metastatic disease. As indicated in Figure 18-5, stage I disease carries a relatively good prognosis as compared with the dismal prognosis of stage IV disease.

Ten-Year Survival Rates in Patients with Melanoma
by Tumor Thickness and Ulceration (n = 4568)[†]

Thickness, mm	Number of patients with		10-year survival rate		
	No ulceration, percent	Ulceration, percent	No ulceration	Ulceration	P value
0.01–1.00	2017 (95.5)	96 (4.5)	92.0	69.1	<0.0001
1.01–2.00	944 (78.8)	255 (21.2)	77.7	62.9	<0.0001
2.01–4.00	500 (57.4)	372 (42.6)	59.5	53.2	0.006
>4.00	146 (38.1)	238 (61.9)	54.5	35.5	0.0006

[†]Modified from Buzaid AC, Ross MI, Balch CM, et al, *J Clin Oncol* 1997;15:1039.

Figure 18-5 • Survival rate by years after diagnosis. Stage I 5-year survival rate: 96–99% for primary lesions <0.76 mm thick; 87–94% for primary lesions 0.76–1.5 mm thick.
Reproduced by permission from Greene FL, Page DL, Fleming ID, et al. *AJCC Cancer Staging Manual.* 6th ed. New York, NY: Springer-Verlag; 2002.

In melanoma, tumor thickness is inversely related to survival and is the single most important prognostic indicator. Historically, there have been two systems for classifying melanomas: the Breslow thickness scale and Clark's level of tumor invasion.

The Breslow scale defines primary melanomas that are <0.76 mm thick as local tumors. These tumors have >90% cure rates after simple excision. Individuals with tumors 0.76 to 4.0 mm thick have a >80% risk of having distant disease and a <50% chance of 5-year survival.

Clark's levels of tumor invasion provides an anatomic description of tumor invasion. The level of tumor invasion can be used for discussing prognosis and planning surgical management (Fig. 18-6).

TNM (tumors, nodes, metastases) staging defines stage 1 tumors as T1 lesions (≤0.76 mm thick) *or* as T2 lesions (0.76–1.50 mm thick) with negative nodes and no metastases. Stage 2 tumors are T3 lesions (1.51–4.00 mm thick) *or* T4 lesions (>4.00 mm thick) with negative nodes and no metastases. Stage 3 tumors have fewer than three regional metastases (N1) and no distant metastases, whereas stage 4 tumors have metastases in skin or subcutaneous tissue, distant lymph node metastases, or visceral metastases.

TREATMENT

Surgical excision is the treatment of choice for primary melanomas. The size of the surgical margin is based on the thickness of the primary lesion (Table 18-1).

■ TABLE 18-1 Suggested Margins for Surgical Excision of Melanoma	
Melanoma Thickness	**Margin**
In situ	5 mm
<1 mm thick	1 cm
>1 mm thick	2 cm

Most tissue defects are primarily closed without skin grafting. If primary biopsy specimens are found to have tumor-negative margins, no further surgical treatment is required. Primary mucosal melanomas have poor outcomes because disease is usually extensive. Nail bed lesions require amputation at the distal interphalangeal joint for finger primaries and the interphalangeal joint for thumb primaries.

Regarding regional disease, the performance of elective regional lymph node dissection for nonpalpable nodes is not routine. The thickness of the primary melanoma is used to predict the chance of regional lymph node metastases. Thin lesions limited to the epidermis have a low likelihood of lymph node metastasis, whereas thick lesions invading the subcutaneous fat have a higher likelihood of spread. Regional lymphadenectomy is usually only performed for thick lesions with a high likelihood of nodal spread.

Due to the morbidity of formal regional lymphadenectomy and to increase the ability of detecting microscopic nodal involvement with minimal

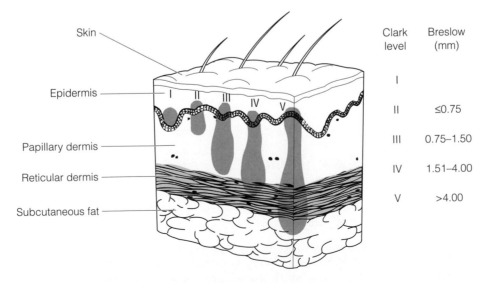

Figure 18-6 • The Clark and Breslow classifications for melanoma.

invasiveness, the technique of sentinal lymph node biopsy (SLNB) was developed. Using lymphoscintigraphy, the sentinel node of the first-order lymph node basin into which the tumor initially drains is identified. In lymphoscintigraphy, technetium (Tc) and a sulfur colloid are circumferentially injected around the primary lesion. The Tc drains via lymphatics to the sentinel node, which is identified using a hand-held scintigrapher. The sentinel node is excised and evaluated microscopically for evidence of metastasis. SLNB is usually considered for lesions >1 mm in thickness.

In metastatic disease, individuals with a single identifiable metastatic lesion may benefit from surgical resection. However, new metastatic lesions usually occur for which surgical intervention is unwarranted. Metastatic sites include skin, lung, brain, bone, liver, and the gastrointestinal tract. Treatment options include surgery, radiation, chemotherapy, and isolated limb perfusion.

PREVENTION

Professional and public education campaigns regarding the dangers of excessive sun exposure, combined with early diagnosis and appropriate surgical removal, increase survival for individuals diagnosed with melanoma.

🔑 18-2 KEY POINTS

1. Melanoma is a potentially lethal skin cancer arising from melanocytes.
2. Melanoma is thought to be caused by ultraviolet light.
3. Melanoma arises mostly from pre-existing moles.
4. The five signs of melanoma are *a*symmetric shape, irregular *b*order, mottled *c*olor, large *d*iameter, and progressive *e*nlargement.
5. The four types of melanoma are superficial spreading, lentigo maligna, acral lentiginous, and nodular.
6. Prognosis for primary tumors is based on tumor thickness: Tumors <0.76 mm have >90% cure rates.
7. Primary tumors require excision margins based on tumor thickness.
8. Nail bed tumors require distal joint amputation.
9. When indicated, sentinal lymph node biopsy confirms regional disease.
10. Sites of metastasis are lung, brain, bone, and the gastrointestinal tract.

SQUAMOUS CELL CARCINOMA

Squamous cell carcinoma (SCC) is the second most common form of skin cancer after BCC. Tumors arise from the skin and the oral and anogenital mucosa. Multiple predisposing factors for development of SCC have been identified.

PATHOGENESIS

The predominant etiology of most SCC is chronic actinic damage that induces the malignant transformation of epidermal keratinocytes. A similar effect is seen with exposure to ionizing radiation (x-rays and gamma rays). In darkly pigmented individuals, however, most lesions arise from sites of chronic inflammation, such as osteomyelitis and chronic tropical ulcerations. Tumors also arise at mucocutaneous interfaces, secondary to tobacco use or human papilloma virus (HPV) infection. Smokers typically present with ulcerating lip and gum or tongue lesions, whereas invasive cancers of the vulva and penis are seen with HPV infection. Anogenital SCC is linked to infection with HPV types 16, 18, 31, 33, and 35. Immunosuppressed or immunocompromised individuals—namely, transplant recipients on immunosuppressive medication or those with human immunodeficiency virus/acquired immunodeficiency syndrome (HIV/AIDS)—have an increased incidence of squamous cell cancer and an elevated rate of metastasis. Rarely, tumors arise from old scars (usually sustained secondary to burn injury), which form so-called Marjolin ulcers or burn scar tumors. As a rule, actinically induced cancers infrequently metastasize, whereas tumors arising from other mechanisms have a significantly higher rate of metastasis (Table 18-2).

■ TABLE 18-2 Predisposing Factors for Developing Squamous Cell Carcinoma

Sunlight exposure
Human papilloma virus infection
Immunosuppression (transplant recipients)
Immunocompromise (HIV infection)
Chronic ulcers
Ionizing radiation (x-rays, gamma rays)
Tobacco use
Scars (burn injury)

HIV, human immunodeficiency virus.

HISTORY

SCC appears as an indurated nodule or plaque, often with ulceration, which has slowly evolved over time. Most lesions are on sun-exposed areas, such as the face, ears, and upper extremities.

PHYSICAL EXAMINATION

Caucasians exhibit pinkish lesions, whereas darker-skinned individuals have hypo- or hyperpigmented lesions (Fig. 18-7). Regional lymphadenopathy occurs in 35% of SCC arising in the lip and mouth. Aberrant keratinization is often seen in SCC, occasionally causing the growth of cutaneous horns. Therefore, the base of a cutaneous horn should always be examined for the presence of squamous cell cancer.

TREATMENT

The preferred treatment is tumor removal by surgical excision. The remaining defect is closed either primarily for smaller lesions or by skin grafting or flap reconstruction for larger lesions. Cryosurgery or cautery/curettage can also be used for small tumors.

PROGNOSIS

The overall cure rate for SCC is 90% after treatment. Tumors other than sun-induced SCC have a higher mortality because of the greater likelihood of metastasis.

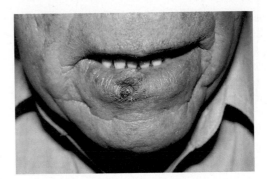

Figure 18-7 • Squamous cell carcinoma. This patient has a nodular, ulcerative lesion on his lip.
From Goodheart HP. *Goodheart's Photoguide of Common Skin Disorders.* 2nd ed. Philadelphia, PA: Lippincott Williams & Wilkins; 2003.

🔑 18-3 KEY POINTS

1. Squamous cell carcinoma (SCC) is the second most common form of skin cancer.
2. SCC is predominantly caused by sunlight exposure.
3. SCC of the oral and anogenital mucosa is associated with tobacco use and human papilloma virus infection.
4. SCC has an increased incidence in immunosuppressed and immunocompromised individuals and exhibits an elevated risk of metastases.
5. SCC may arise in old burn scars as Marjolin ulcers or burn scar carcinoma.
6. SCC may arise in sites of chronic inflammation, such as osteomyelitis and chronic ulcers.
7. SCC typically appears as an indurated nodule or plaque, often with ulceration.
8. Treatment consists of surgical excision.
9. Overall cure rate is 90%.

References

Acarturk TO, Edington H. Nonmelanoma skin cancer. *Clin Plast Surg.* 2005;32(2):237–248.

Aloia TA, Gershenwald JE. Management of early-stage cutaneous melanoma. *Curr Probl Surg.* 2005;42(7):460–534.

Chapter

19 Small Intestine

ANATOMY AND PHYSIOLOGY

The small intestine comprises the duodenum, jejunum, and ileum and extends from the pylorus proximally to the cecum distally. Its main function is to digest and absorb nutrients. Absorption is achieved by the large surface area of the small intestine, secondary to its long length and extensive mucosal projections of villi and microvilli. A broad-based mesentery suspends the small intestine from the posterior abdominal wall once the retroperitoneal duodenum emerges at the ligament of Treitz and becomes the jejunum. Arterial blood is supplied from branches of the superior mesenteric artery, and venous drainage is via the superior mesenteric vein. The mucosa has sequential circular folds called *plicae circulares*. The plicae circulares are more numerous in the proximal bowel than in the distal bowel. The mucosal villi and microvilli create the surface through which carbohydrates, fats, proteins, and electrolytes are absorbed (Figs. 19-1 and 19-2).

SMALL BOWEL OBSTRUCTION

Although the etiology of small bowel obstruction (SBO) is varied, the presentation of this disorder is usually quite consistent because of a common mechanism. Obstruction of the small bowel lumen causes progressive proximal accumulation of intraluminal fluids and gas. Peristalsis continues to transport swallowed air and secreted intestinal fluid through the bowel proximal to the obstruction, resulting in small bowel dilation and eventual abdominal distention. Depending on the location of the obstruction, vomiting occurs early in proximal obstruction and later in more distal blockage (Fig. 19-3). Crampy abdominal pain initially occurs as active proximal peristalsis exacerbates bowel dilation. With progressive bowel wall edema and luminal dilation, however, peristaltic activity decreases and abdominal pain lessens. At presentation, patients exhibit abdominal distention and complain of mild diffuse abdominal pain.

ETIOLOGY

The first and second most common causes of SBO are adhesions and hernias (Table 19-1). Most adhesions are caused by postoperative internal scar formation. Discovering the actual mechanism of obstruction is also important, because it relates to the possibility of vascular compromise and bowel ischemia. For example, a closed-loop obstruction caused by volvulus with torsion is at high risk for vascular compromise. This is often seen when a loop of small bowel twists around an adhesion.

A second mechanism causing bowel ischemia is incarceration in a fixed space. Incarceration and subsequent strangulation impede venous return, causing edema and eventual bowel infarction. Other mechanisms of obstruction that rarely compromise vascular flow are obstruction of the bowel lumen by a gallstone or bezoar and intussusception caused by an intramural or mucosal lesion at the leading edge.

HISTORY

Patients usually present with complaints of intermittent crampy abdominal pain, abdominal distention, obstipation, nausea, and vomiting. Vomiting of feculent material usually occurs later in the course of obstruction. Constant localizable pain or pain out of

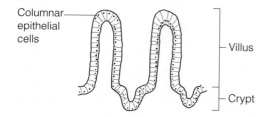

Columnar epithelial cells

Villus

Crypt

Figure 19-1 • Structure of small intestinal villi.

proportion to physical findings may indicate ischemic bowel and is a clear indication for urgent surgical exploration.

PHYSICAL EXAMINATION

A distended abdomen with diffuse midabdominal tenderness to palpation is usually found on physical examination. Typically, there are no signs of peritonitis. If constant localized tenderness is apparent, ischemia and gangrene must be suspected. An essential aspect of the examination is to check for abdominal wall hernias, especially in postsurgical patients. Elevation in temperature should not be present in uncomplicated cases. Tachycardia may be present from hypovolemia secondary to persistent vomiting or from toxemia caused by intestinal gangrene.

DIAGNOSTIC EVALUATION

Upright radiographs classically demonstrate distended loops of small bowel with multiple air–fluid interfaces. Occasionally, the radiograph shows the etiology of the obstruction, the site of obstruction, and whether the obstruction is partial or complete. Free air indicates perforation, whereas biliary gas and an opacity near the ileocecal valve indicate gallstone ileus.

TREATMENT

Initial treatment consists of nasogastric decompression to relieve proximal gastrointestinal distention and associated nausea and vomiting. Fluid resuscitation follows, because patients are usually intravascularly depleted from persistent vomiting.

The decision to operate is based on the nature of the obstruction and the patient's condition. If ischemia or perforation is suspected, immediate operation is necessary. Otherwise, patients can be observed with serial physical examinations and radiographs for evidence of resolution. If the patient's condition worsens or fails to improve with supportive therapy, operative intervention is clearly indicated.

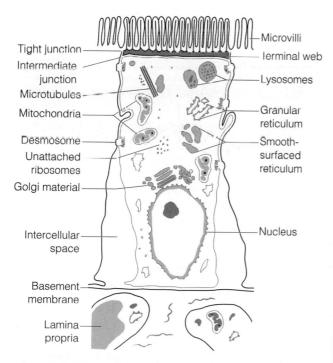

Tight junction
Intermediate junction
Microtubules
Mitochondria
Desmosome
Unattached ribosomes
Golgi material
Intercellular space
Basement membrane
Lamina propria

Microvilli
Terminal web
Lysosomes
Granular reticulum
Smooth-surfaced reticulum
Nucleus

Figure 19-2 • Diagram of a columnar epithelial intestinal absorptive cell with luminal microvilli.

🔑 19-1 KEY POINTS

1. Small bowel obstruction is commonly caused by adhesions and hernias.
2. Patients complain of progressive abdominal distention, diffuse crampy abdominal pain, nausea, and vomiting.
3. Infarction occurs with closed-loop obstruction and with strangulation. Patients with peritonitis require immediate surgery.
4. Many patients are successfully managed with supportive therapy alone. Surgery is indicated if the obstruction fails to resolve spontaneously.
5. Distended small bowel loops with multiple air–fluid interfaces are seen on x-ray. Biliary gas and a right lower quadrant opacity indicate gallstone ileus.

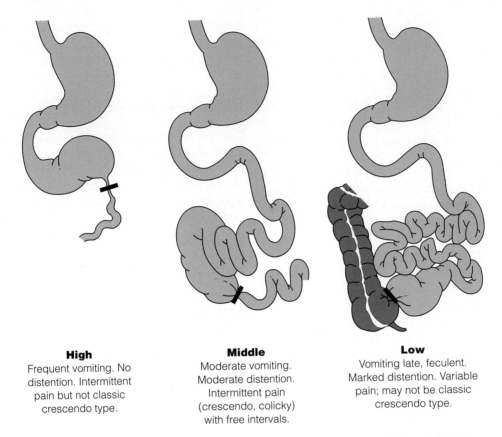

High
Frequent vomiting. No distention. Intermittent pain but not classic crescendo type.

Middle
Moderate vomiting. Moderate distention. Intermittent pain (crescendo, colicky) with free intervals.

Low
Vomiting late, feculent. Marked distention. Variable pain; may not be classic crescendo type.

Figure 19-3 • Variable manifestations of small bowel obstruction depend on the level of blockage.

CROHN DISEASE

Crohn disease is a transmural inflammatory disease that may affect any part of the gastrointestinal tract, from the mouth to the anus. Ileal involvement is most common. The disease is characterized by skip lesions that involve discontinuous segments of abnormal mucosa. Granulomata are usually seen microscopically, but not always. Areas of inflammation are often associated with fibrotic strictures, enterocutaneous fistulae, and intra-abdominal abscesses, all of which usually require surgical intervention.

EPIDEMIOLOGY

Crohn disease occurs throughout the world, although the actual incidence exhibits a geographic and ethnic variability. The incidence in the United States is approximately 10 times that of Japan. Ashkenazi Jews have a far higher incidence of disease than do African Americans.

■ TABLE 19-1 Causes of Small Bowel Obstruction
Adhesions
Hernias—abdominal wall, internal
Neoplasms—primary, metastatic
Obturation/strictures—ischemia, radiation, Crohn disease, gallstone, bezoar
Intussusception
Meckel diverticulum
Volvulus
Superior mesenteric artery syndrome
Intramural hematoma

ETIOLOGY

The etiology of Crohn disease remains unknown. Because of the presence of granulomata, mycobacterial infection has been postulated as the causative agent. Recent investigations with *Mycobacterium paratuberculosis* have proved inconclusive. An immunologic basis for the disease has also been advanced; however, although humoral and cellular immune responses are involved in disease pathogenesis, no specific immunologic disturbance has been identified.

PATHOLOGY

The small intestine is affected in at least 70% of all patients with Crohn disease. The ileum is typically diseased, with frequent right colon involvement. On gross inspection, the serosal surface of the bowel is hypervascular and the mesentery characteristically shows signs of "creeping fat." The bowel walls are edematous and fibrotic. The mucosa has a cobblestone appearance, with varying degrees of associated mucosal ulceration. Histologically, a chronic lymphocytic infiltrate in an inflamed mucosa and submucosa is seen. Fissure ulcers penetrate deep into the mucosa and are often associated with granulomata and multinucleated giant cells. Granulomata are seen more frequently in distal tissues, which explains why granulomata are seen more often in colonic disease than in ileal disease.

HISTORY

Patients with Crohn disease of the small bowel present complaining of diarrhea, abdominal pain, anorexia, nausea, and weight loss. The diarrhea is usually loose and watery without frank blood. Dull abdominal pain is usually in the right iliac fossa or periumbilical region. Children often present with symptoms of malaise and have noticeable growth failure. Strictures may cause partial SBO, resulting in bacterial overgrowth and subsequent steatorrhea, flatus, and bloating.

PHYSICAL EXAMINATION

Patients may appear to be either generally healthy or may have significant cachexia. Abdominal examination may reveal right iliac fossa tenderness. In acutely ill patients, a palpable abdominal mass may be present, indicating abscess formation. Enterocutaneous fistulae may be present. Oral examination may reveal evidence of mucosal ulceration, whereas perianal inspection may show skin tags, fissures, or fistulae. Extraintestinal manifestations include erythema nodosum, pyoderma gangrenosum, ankylosing spondylitis, and uveitis.

DIAGNOSTIC EVALUATION

Blood studies often show a mild iron-deficiency anemia and a depressed albumin level. If hypoalbuminemia is severe, peripheral edema may be present.

Small intestine Crohn disease is diagnosed by barium-contrast enteroclysis. This small intestine enema technique provides better mucosal definition than do standard small bowel follow-through studies. This technique illustrates aphthoid ulcers, strictures, fissures, bowel wall thickening, and fistulae. Fistulograms are helpful to define existing fistula tracks, and computed tomography (CT) can localize abscesses. Once radiographic evidence of disease is found, colonoscopy should be performed to evaluate the colonic mucosa and to obtain biopsies of the terminal ileum.

DIFFERENTIAL DIAGNOSIS

In addition to the diagnosis of Crohn disease, one should consider the possibility of acute appendicitis, *Yersinia* infection, lymphoma, intestinal tuberculosis, and Behçet disease.

COMPLICATIONS

Crohn disease carries a high morbidity and low mortality. Small bowel strictures, secondary to inflammation, and fibrosis are common complications that present as obstructions. Fistulae from small bowel to adjacent loops of small bowel, large bowel, bladder, vagina, or skin also occur. Ileal Crohn disease can result in gallstone formation because of the interruption of the enterohepatic circulation of bile salts. Kidney stones may also form because of hyperoxaluria. Normally, calcium and oxalate bind in the intestine and are excreted in the feces. With ileal Crohn disease, steatorrhea causes ingested fat to bind intraluminal calcium, thus allowing free oxalate to be absorbed. Finally, adenocarcinoma is a rare complication that usually arises in the ileum.

TREATMENT

Mild disease can be controlled with a 4- to 6-week course of sulfasalazine or mesalazine. Alternatively, oral corticosteroids can be used with equivalent results. Metronidazole may also be useful. Patients with bile salt-induced diarrhea after ileal resection may benefit from cholestyramine.

Severe disease is treated with hospitalization, bowel rest, hydration, intravenous nutrition, steroids,

TABLE 19-2 Indications for Surgery in Crohn Disease

Stenosis with obstructive symptoms

Fistula

Abscess

Perforation

Bleeding

and metronidazole. Patients with chronic active disease may benefit from a course of 6-mercaptopurine.

Surgery for Crohn disease should only be performed for complications of the disease (Table 19-2). Operation should be conservative and should address only the presenting indication, using gentle surgical technique. Resections should be avoided, as overly aggressive intervention can produce surgically induced short bowel syndrome and malnutrition. Some common surgical problems encountered in Crohn disease and its treatments include ileocolic disease, which is managed by conservative ileocecal resection to grossly normal margins (Fig. 19-4); stricture, managed by stricturoplasty, which entails incising the antimesenteric border of the stricture along the intestinal long axis and then closing the enterotomy transversely (Fig. 19-5); and abscess/fistula, which is managed by

open or percutaneous drainage of the abscess and resection of the small bowel segment responsible for initiating the fistula with primary anastomosis (Fig. 19-6).

🔑 19-2 KEY POINTS

1. Crohn disease is a transmural inflammatory process that affects any part of the gastrointestinal tract, from the mouth to the anus.
2. The ileum is most commonly involved. Discontinuous mucosal skip lesions are seen macroscopically, with associated granulomata seen microscopically.
3. Extraintestinal manifestations include erythema nodosum, pyoderma gangrenosum, ankylosing spondylitis, and uveitis.
4. Ileal disease may cause gallstones and kidney stones by interrupting the enterohepatic circulation of bile salts and by increasing gastrointestinal oxalate absorption, respectively.

MECKEL DIVERTICULUM

This most common congenital anomaly of the small intestine is an antimesenteric remnant arising from a failure of vitelline duct obliteration during embryonic

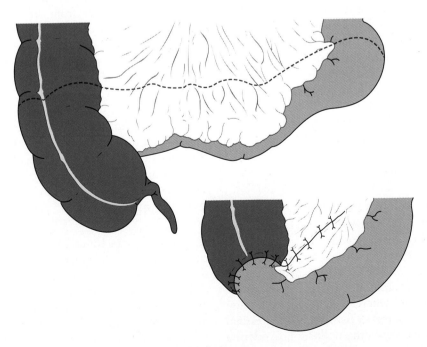

Figure 19-4 • Ileocecal resection for Crohn disease.

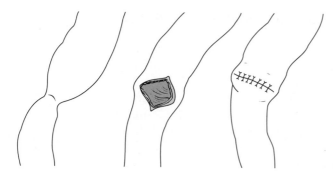

Figure 19-5 • Stricturoplasty of a localized stricture with transverse closure.

development. Meckel diverticula are true diverticula affecting all three intestinal muscle layers. Diverticula are usually <12 cm in length and are found within 100 cm of the ileocecal valve.

Associated abnormalities of the vitelline duct depend on the degree of duct obliteration that occurs during development. Complete ductal obliteration leaves a thin fibrous band connecting ileum to umbilicus, whereas complete duct persistence results in a patent ileoumbilical fistula. Partial obstruction results in cyst or blind sinus formation (Fig. 19-7). Heterotopic tissue (gastric, pancreatic) is found in 30% to 50% of diverticula.

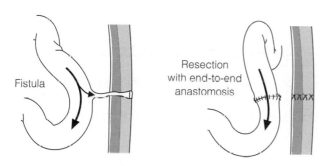

Figure 19-6 • Fistula resection with end-to-end anastomosis.

In the United States, Meckel diverticulum is associated with the "rule of 2s": It occurs in 2% of the population, is located within 2 ft of the ileocecal valve, is usually 2 in. long, contains two types of heterotopic tissue (gastric, pancreatic, duodenal, or intestinal), and is the most common cause of rectal bleeding in infants under the age of 2.

COMPLICATIONS

Bleeding within the diverticulum may occur from peptic ulceration arising from heterotopic gastric mucosa. In infants, Meckel diverticulum is the most common cause of major lower gastrointestinal bleeding.

Bowel obstruction may result from one of two mechanisms: Intussusception can occur when an inverted diverticulum functions as a lead point, or small bowel volvulus can occur around a fixed obliterated vitelline duct extending from the ileum to the umbilicus.

DIAGNOSTIC EVALUATION

For Meckel diverticula containing heterotopic gastric mucosa, the technetium (Tc)-99 scan is helpful for diagnosis: Pertechnetate anions are taken up by ectopic gastric parietal cells and indicate diverticulum location. Diverticula that do not contain heterotopic gastric tissue can occasionally be visualized using standard barium-contrast studies.

TREATMENT

Definitive treatment for Meckel diverticulum complications is surgical resection. In adult patients incidentally found to have an asymptomatic Meckel diverticulum during laparotomy, the diverticulum should be left in situ, as the chance of producing surgical

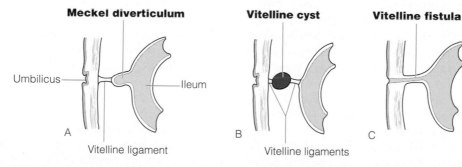

Figure 19-7 • Vitelline duct remnants.

morbidity and mortality are 23 and 5 times higher for resection than when only symptomatic diverticula are removed.

⚷ 19-3 KEY POINTS

1. Meckel diverticulum is the most common congenital abnormality of the small intestine and arises from a failure of vitelline duct obliteration.
2. It is a true diverticulum and may contain heterotopic gastric and pancreatic tissue.
3. Peptic ulceration, the most common cause of major lower gastrointestinal bleeding in infants, may develop in patients with Meckel diverticulum.
4. Incidentally found Meckel diverticula should be left in situ.

SMALL BOWEL TUMORS

Tumors of the small bowel are rare, accounting for 1% to 5% of all gastrointestinal tumors. Most tumors are benign. Common benign neoplasms of the small bowel include tubular and villous adenomas, lipomas, leiomyomas, and hemangiomas. Telangiectasias of Rendu-Osler-Weber syndrome, neurofibromas of neurofibromatosis, hamartomatous polyps of Peutz-Jeghers syndrome, and heterotopic tissue as in Meckel diverticulum are also found. Possible explanations for this lack of malignancy include short exposure to ingested carcinogens secondary to rapid transit time, low bacterial counts resulting in fewer endogenously produced carcinogens, and the intraluminal secretion of immunoglobulin A by small bowel mucosa.

Benign lesions are usually asymptomatic and are incidental findings. Of symptomatic lesions, obstruction is the most common presentation, followed by hemorrhage. In the workup of gastrointestinal bleeding, however, unless other evidence exists, small bowel lesions should be low on the list of differential diagnoses, because >90% of bleeding lesions occur between the esophagus and distal duodenum and between the ileocecal valve and anus. Small bowel lesions should be suspected if careful skin examination reveals café-au-lait spots (neurofibromatosis), telangiectasia (Rendu-Osler-Weber syndrome), or mucocutaneous pigmentation (Peutz-Jeghers syndrome).

Malignant tumors of the small bowel typically present with obstruction or bleeding. The four major malignant tumors are adenocarcinoma, gastrointestinal stromal tumors, carcinoid, and lymphoma.

DIAGNOSTIC EVALUATION

Visual endoscopic identification of small bowel tumors is usually possible for lesions of the proximal duodenum and terminal ileum. The remainder of the small bowel requires examination by barium-contrast studies. For larger lesions, CT may be helpful.

In situations involving active hemorrhage, Tc-99 sulfur colloid or Tc-99–labeled red blood cell studies may show the bleeding site. However, a bleeding rate of 1 mL per minute is required for accurate localization.

When available diagnostic modalities are insufficient, exploratory laparotomy may be necessary. In addition to external inspection at laparotomy, operative endoscopy can be used for intraluminal evaluation.

⚷ 19-4 KEY POINTS

1. Small bowel tumors are rare and usually benign.
2. Tumors commonly present as small bowel obstructions.
3. Benign tumors include adenomas, lipomas, leiomyomas, and hemangiomas.
4. Malignant tumors include adenocarcinoma, gastrointestinal stromal tumors, carcinoid, and lymphoma.

CARCINOID TUMORS

Carcinoid tumors are the most common endocrine tumors of the gastrointestinal tract, constituting more than half of all such lesions. They account for up to 30% of all small bowel tumors. Carcinoid tumors arise from neuroendocrine enterochromaffin cells. Hence, tumors can secrete serotonin and other humoral substances, such as histamine, dopamine, tachykinins, peptides, and prostaglandins. The metabolite of serotonin, 5-hydroxyindoleacetic acid (5-HIAA), is excreted in the urine and is easily detected.

All carcinoids are considered malignant due to their potential for invasion and metastasis. Patients with metastatic disease manifest the carcinoid syndrome, which consists of the systemic effects (flushing, diarrhea, sweating, and wheezing) of secreted vasoactive substances. Presence of the carcinoid syndrome indicates hepatic metastasis, because systemic effects occur when venous drainage from a tumor escapes hepatic metabolism of vasoactive substances.

Approximately 85% of carcinoid tumors are found in the intestine; of these, about 50% are found in the appendix, making it the most common site of occurrence, followed by the ileum, jejunum, rectum, and duodenum. Other sites of disease include the lungs and occasionally the pancreas and biliary tract. Appendiceal carcinoids rarely metastasize, whereas lesions of the ileum have the highest association with carcinoid syndrome. Jejunoileal carcinoids are frequently multicentric.

HISTORY

The clinical presentation of patients with carcinoid tumors differs depending on tumor location. Primary tumors may present as SBO, because tumors can incite an intense local fibrosis of the bowel that causes angulation and kinking of the involved segment. As noted, metastatic disease with hepatic spread manifests as the carcinoid syndrome. Occult primary lesions do not cause systemic effects because 5-hydroxytryptamine (serotonin) is metabolized by the liver. Other presenting symptoms can include abdominal pain, upper intestinal or rectal bleeding, intussusception, weight loss, or a palpable abdominal mass.

DIAGNOSTIC EVALUATION

Laboratory studies should include plasma and urine analysis to evaluate for elevated levels of plasma serotonin and urinary 5-HIAA. Barium-contrast studies are also useful for diagnosing carcinoid tumors. Barium enemas can demonstrate lesions of the rectum and large bowel, whereas small bowel enteroclysis may show a discrete lesion or a stricture secondary to fibrosis. Because primary tumors are usually small, CT is usually helpful only for detecting hepatic metastases. Colonoscopy can show tumors from the terminal ileum to the rectum.

Because neuroendocrine tumors often express functional receptors, radiolabeled octreotide imaging can be useful in detecting occult disease. Octreotide scanning is based on physiologic function, rather than on detectable anatomic alterations, and may have better diagnostic sensitivity than conventional imaging modalities.

TREATMENT

Surgical resection of the primary tumor is always undertaken, even in cases of metastatic disease. If the tumor is left in situ, bowel obstruction and intussusception ultimately result. At laparotomy, adequate bowel and mesenteric margins must be obtained, as with any cancer operation. Depending on tumor size and the degree of spread, lesions can be treated with simple local excision for small primaries to wide en bloc resection for metastatic disease.

Patients who have carcinoid syndrome can achieve symptomatic relief with subcutaneous injections of somatostatin analogues (e.g., octreotide). Induction with general anesthesia may provoke a life-threatening carcinoid crisis characterized by hypotension, flushing, tachycardia, and arrhythmias. Intravenous somatostatin or octreotide rapidly reverse the crisis.

PROGNOSIS

Carcinoid tumors are relatively indolent, slow-growing neoplasms. Prognosis for patients with carcinoid tumors is directly related to the size of the primary tumor and to the presence of metastasis.

For noninvasive lesions of the appendix and rectum <2 cm in size, the 5-year survival rate nears 100%. As the tumor size increases, the survival rate decreases. The presence of muscle wall invasion and positive lymph nodes are poor prognostic signs.

Patients with hepatic metastases have an average survival of approximately 3 years. Liver lesions are usually multiple. Because incapacitating symptoms of the carcinoid syndrome are proportional to tumor bulk, cytoreductive surgery can ameliorate symptoms, as well as prolong survival. Nonsurgical palliation is achieved with somatostatin analogue therapy or chemoembolization of the tumor.

🔑 19-5 KEY POINTS

1. Carcinoid tumors are the most common endocrine tumors of the gastrointestinal tract.
2. Carcinoid tumors most frequently occur in the appendix.
3. All carcinoid tumors are considered malignant because of their potential for invasion and metastasis.
4. Carcinoid tumors secrete serotonin, which is broken down in the liver to the metabolite 5-hydroxyindoleacetic acid, which is, in turn, excreted in the urine.
5. Carcinoid syndrome manifests as flushing, diarrhea, sweating, and wheezing and is caused by the systemic effects of secreted vasoactive substances.
6. Carcinoid syndrome invariably indicates hepatic metastases, because vasoactive substances have escaped hepatic metabolism.
7. Carcinoid syndrome is treated with somatostatin analogues and chemoembolization to provide symptomatic relief.

References

Akerstrom G. Management of midgut carcinoids. *J Surg Oncol*. 2005;89(3):161–169.

Ottinger LW. Small bowel obstruction. In: Morris PJ, Wood WC. *Oxford Textbook of Surgery*. New York, NY: Oxford University Press; 1994:961–964.

Podolsky, DK. Inflammatory bowel diesease. *N Eng J Med*. 2002;347:417–429.

Stomach and Duodenum

The stomach and duodenum are discussed as a single unit because they are anatomically contiguous structures, share an interrelated physiology, and have similar disease processes. Peptic ulceration is the most common inflammatory disorder of the gastrointestinal tract and is responsible for significant disability. The stomach and duodenum are principally affected by peptic ulceration.

ANATOMY

The stomach is divided into the fundus, body, and antrum (Fig. 20-1). The fundus is the superior dome of the stomach; the body extends from the fundus to the angle of the stomach (incisura angularis), located on the lesser curvature; and the antrum extends from the body to the pylorus. Hydrochloric acid secreting parietal cells are found in the fundus, pepsinogen-secreting chief cells are found in the proximal stomach, and gastrin-secreting G cells are found in the antrum.

Six arterial sources supply blood to the stomach: the left and right gastric arteries to the lesser curvature; the left and right gastroepiploic arteries to the greater curvature; the short gastric arteries, branching from the splenic artery to supply the fundus; and the gastroduodenal artery, branching to the pylorus (Fig. 20-2). The vagus nerve supplies parasympathetic innervation via the anterior left and posterior right trunks. These nerves stimulate gastric motility and the secretion of pepsinogen and hydrochloric acid.

The duodenum is divided into four portions (Fig. 20-3). The first portion begins at the pylorus and includes the duodenal bulb. The ampulla of Vater, through which the common bile duct and pancreatic duct drain, is located in the medial wall of the descending second portion of the duodenum. The transverse third portion is traversed anteriorly by the superior mesenteric vessels. The ascending fourth portion terminates at the ligament of Treitz, which defines the duodenal–jejunal junction. The arterial supply to the duodenum is via the superior pancreaticoduodenal artery, which arises from the gastroduodenal artery, and via the inferior pancreaticoduodenal artery, which arises from the superior mesenteric artery.

GASTRIC AND DUODENAL ULCERATION

PATHOGENESIS

The etiology of benign peptic gastric and duodenal ulceration involves a compromised mucosal surface undergoing acid-peptic digestion. Substances that alter mucosal defenses include nonsteroidal anti-inflammatory drugs (NSAIDs), alcohol, and tobacco use. Alcohol directly attacks the mucosa, NSAIDs alter prostaglandin synthesis, and smoking restricts mucosal vascular perfusion. The most important recent advance in understanding the pathogenesis of peptic ulceration is the realization that infestation with the organism *Helicobacter pylori* plays an important role in gastric and duodenal ulceration. The 2005 Nobel Prize in medicine was awarded to Drs. Marshall and Warren of Australia "for their discovery of the bacterium *Helicobacter pylori* and its role in gastritis and peptic ulcer disease."

HISTORY

Patients typically present complaining of epigastric pain relieved by food or antacids. Sensations of fullness and mild nausea are common, but vomiting is rare unless pyloric obstruction is present secondary to scarring. Physical examination is often benign except for occasional epigastric tenderness.

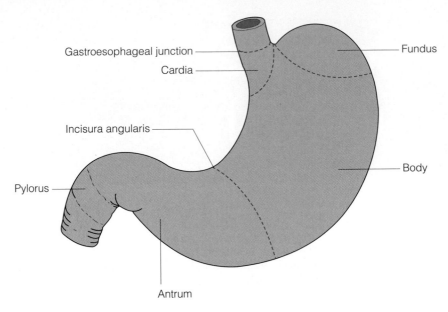

Figure 20-1 • Anatomy of the stomach.

DIAGNOSTIC EVALUATION

The radiographic evaluation of peptic ulcers entails barium studies that reveal evidence of crater deformities at areas of ulceration. Serum testing determines whether there are antibodies to *H. pylori* and breath testing confirms infection.

Definitive diagnosis is made by direct visualization of the ulcer using endoscopy. For nonhealing gastric ulcers refractory to medical therapy, it is extremely

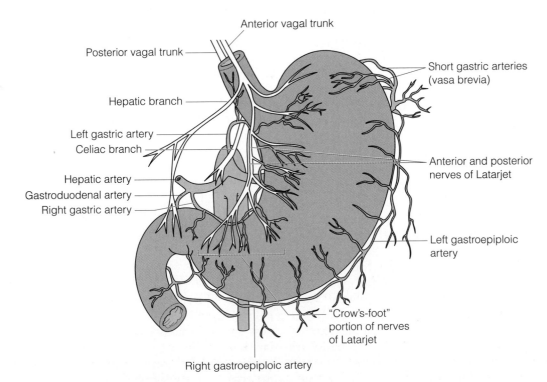

Figure 20-2 • Blood supply and parasympathetic innervation of the stomach and duodenum.

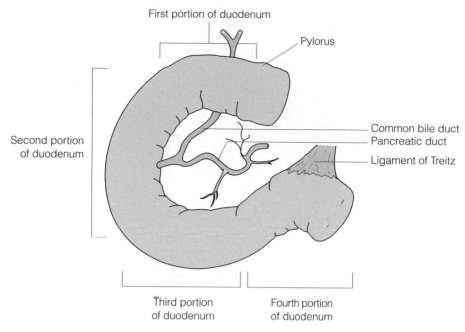

Figure 20-3 • Anatomy of the duodenum.

important that biopsy of the ulcer be performed to rule out gastric carcinoma. Duodenal ulcers are rarely malignant.

TREATMENT

Medical treatment is similar for gastric and duodenal ulceration. The goals of medical therapy are to decrease production of or neutralize stomach acid and to enhance mucosal protection against acid attack. Medications include antacids (CaCO3), H2-blockers (cimetidine, ranitidine), mucosal coating agents (sucralfate), prostaglandins (misoprostol), and proton-pump inhibitors (omeprazole). If *H. pylori* is present, treatment with oral antibiotics is associated with a 90% eradication rate. Treatment regimens may consist of tetracycline/metronidazole/bismuth subsalicylate, amoxicillin/metronidazole/ranitidine, or other combinations.

Due to the advent of proton-pump inhibitors (PPI) and the increased understanding of the role *H. pylori* plays in peptic ulceration, operations for ulcer disease have become infrequent. Indications for surgical treatment in the acute setting are either perforation or massive bleeding. Indications for elective operation are a chronic nonhealing ulcer after medical therapy or gastric outlet obstruction. The operation chosen must address the indication for which the procedure

is performed. Historically, before the era of PPIs and *H. pylori*, the goal of surgery was to permanently reduce acid secretion by removing the entire antrum. In most instances, vagotomy and distal gastrectomy (antrectomy), with Billroth I or II anastomosis, fulfilled these criteria (Figs. 20-4 and 20-5). Because denervation of the stomach by truncal vagotomy alters normal patterns of gastric motility and causes gastric atony, surgical drainage procedures are required afterward to ensure satisfactory gastric emptying. Today, most cases of perforation are treated with closure of the defect with omental patch, and cases of bleeding are treated with suture ligation of the bleeding vessel.

🔑 20-1 KEY POINTS

1. Peptic ulceration involves a compromised mucosal surface undergoing acid-peptic digestion.
2. Causes include *Helicobacter pylori* infection, non-steroidal anti-inflammatory drugs, alcohol, and tobacco use, all of which alter mucosal defenses.
3. Treatment consists of decreasing stomach acidity and enhancing mucosal protection. *H. pylori* is eradicated with oral antibiotic therapy.
4. Peptic ulceration is treated surgically for perforation, massive bleeding, gastric outlet obstruction, and a nonhealing ulcer.

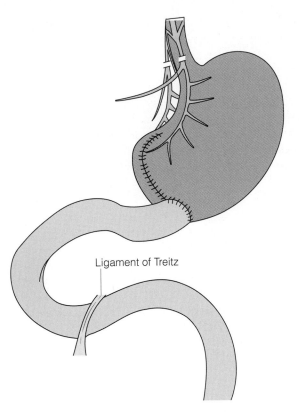

Figure 20-4 • Vagotomy and antrectomy with Billroth I anastomosis.

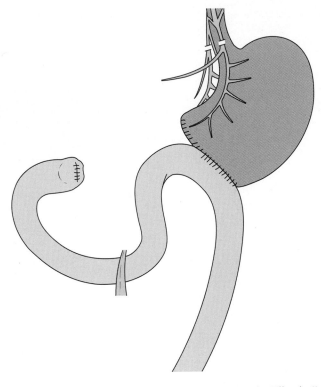

Figure 20-5 • Vagotomy and antrectomy with Billroth II anastomosis.

STRESS GASTRITIS AND ULCERATION

PATHOGENESIS

Critically ill patients subjected to severe physiologic stress, often in the intensive care unit setting, are at risk for developing gastroduodenal mucosal erosion that can progress to ulceration. The commonly accepted etiology of stress gastritis and ulceration is mucosal ischemia induced by an episode of hypotension from hemorrhage, sepsis, hypovolemia, or cardiac dysfunction. Ischemia disrupts cellular mechanisms of mucosal protection, resulting in mucosal acidification and superficial erosion. Areas of erosion may coalesce and form superficial ulcers. Stress ulcers may be seen throughout the stomach and proximal duodenum.

HISTORY

Patients are usually critically ill and have a recent history of hypotension. Massive upper gastrointestinal bleeding is the usual finding.

DIAGNOSTIC EVALUATION

Sites of hemorrhage can be identified by endoscopy.

TREATMENT

Endoscopy can often control bleeding by either electrocoagulation or photocoagulation. Persistent or recurrent bleeding unresponsive to endoscopic techniques requires surgical intervention. Depending on the circumstances, operations for control of bleeding stress gastritis or ulcer require oversewing of the bleeding vessel. Usually, vagotomy is also performed to reduce acid secretion. In many cases, because bleeding is often diffuse and cannot be controlled by simple suture ligation, partial or total gastrectomy is performed.

PREVENTION

Prevention of stress ulceration involves maintaining blood pressure, tissue perfusion, and acid-base stability, as well as decreasing acid production while bolstering mucosal protection. The incidence of life-threatening hemorrhagic gastritis has decreased as intravenous H2-blocker therapy and oral cytoprotectants have been introduced to the intensive care setting.

CUSHING ULCER

Distinct from stress gastritis, Cushing ulcers are seen in patients with intracranial pathology (e.g., tumors, head injury). Ulcers are single and deep and may involve the esophagus, stomach, and duodenum. Because of the depth of ulceration, perforation is a common complication. Neuronally mediated acid hypersecretion is thought to be the main etiology of Cushing ulcer.

ZOLLINGER-ELLISON SYNDROME AND GASTRINOMAS

PATHOGENESIS

Zollinger-Ellison syndrome occurs in patients with severe peptic ulceration and evidence of a gastrinoma (non–B cell pancreatic tumor). Peptic ulceration results from the production of large volumes of highly acidic gastric secretions due to elevated serum gastrin levels. Ninety percent of gastrinomas are found in the "gastrinoma triangle," defined by the junction of the cystic duct and the common bile duct, the junction of the second and third portions of the duodenum, and the junction of the neck and body of the pancreas.

HISTORY

Gastrin-secreting tumors produce a clinical picture of epigastric pain, weight loss, vomiting, and severe diarrhea.

DIAGNOSTIC EVALUATION

Diagnosis is confirmed by the secretin-stimulation test, in which the injection of intravenous secretin elevates serum gastrin levels to at least 200 pg/mL. Once diagnosed, tumor localization is performed by magnetic resonance imaging, abdominal ultrasound, computed tomography (CT), selective abdominal angiography, or selective venous sampling.

TREATMENT

Acid hypersecretion can be controlled medically with H2 blockade and PPI. Somatostatin analogues (octreotide) have been found to be effective in decreasing tumor secretion of gastrin and in controlling the growth of tumor metastases.

Gastrinoma is a curable disease, despite the malignant nature of most tumors. Complete resection of tumors results in a near 100% 10-year survival rate. Incomplete resection or unresectability carries <50% 10-year survival rate. When simple excision or enucleation for cure is not feasible, an attempt is made to prolong survival by debulking and performing lymph node dissection to reduce tumor burden and acid hypersecretion.

STOMACH CANCER

Despite the decreasing incidence of gastric carcinoma in Western populations during the past decades, patient survival has not improved. In the United States, fewer than 10% of patients with stomach cancer survive 5 years. Illustrative of geographic variation, stomach cancer is endemic in Japan. Because of the high incidence of disease, mass screening programs are able to detect early-stage lesions, which accounts for a 50% overall survival rate at 5 years.

RISK FACTORS

Environmental and dietary factors are thought to influence the development of gastric cancer. Smoked fish and meats contain benzopyrene, a probable carcinogen to gastric mucosa. Nitrosamines are known carcinogens that are formed by the conversion of dietary nitrogen to nitrosamines in the gastrointestinal tract by bacterial metabolism. Atrophic gastritis, as seen in patients with hypogammaglobulinemia and pernicious anemia, is considered to be a premalignant condition for developing gastric cancer, because high gastric pH encourages bacterial growth. Chronic atrophic gastritis results in achlorhydria, and 75% of patients with gastric cancer are achlorhydric.

PATHOLOGY

Most tumors are adenocarcinomas, and spread is via lymphatics, venous drainage, and direct extension. Most tumors are located in the antral prepyloric region.

Gastric tumors can be typed according to gross appearance. Polypoid fungating nodular tumors are usually well differentiated and carry a relatively good prognosis after surgery. Ulcerating or penetrating tumors are the most common and are often mistaken for benign peptic ulcers because of their sessile nature. Superficial spreading lesions diffusely infiltrate through mucosa and submucosa and have a poor prognosis because most are metastatic at the time of diagnosis.

The pathologic staging of gastric cancer is based on depth of tumor invasion and lymph node status. The pathologic stage of a specific tumor correlates closely with survival (Fig. 20-6).

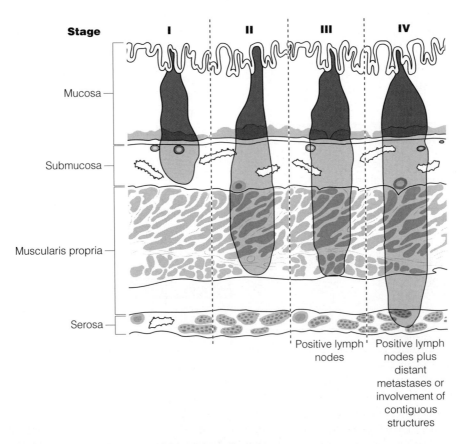

Figure 20-6 • Staging system for gastric carcinoma.

HISTORY

Patients with gastric cancer usually give a history of vague and nonspecific symptoms. Upper abdominal discomfort, dyspepsia, early satiety, belching, weight loss, anorexia, nausea, vomiting, hematemesis, or melena is common. Definite symptoms do not occur until tumor growth causes luminal obstruction, tumor infiltration results in gastric dysmotility, or erosion causes bleeding. By the time of diagnosis, tumors are usually unresectable. Later symptoms indicative of metastatic disease are abdominal distention due to ascites, from hepatic or peritoneal metastases, and dyspnea and pleural effusions, from pulmonary metastases.

PHYSICAL EXAMINATION

Few findings are noted on physical examination, except in advanced disease. A firm, nontender, mobile epigastric mass can be palpated, and hepatomegaly with ascites may be present. Other distant signs of metastatic disease include Virchow supraclavicular sentinel node, Sister Joseph umbilical node, and Blumer shelf on rectal examination.

DIAGNOSTIC EVALUATION

Anemia is often found on routine blood studies. The anemia is usually hypochromic and microcytic secondary to iron deficiency. Stool is often positive for occult blood.

In recent years, upper endoscopy has replaced the barium-contrast upper gastrointestinal study as the imaging modality of choice. Endoscopy allows direct visualization and biopsy of the tumor. At least four biopsies should be made of the lesion. With ten biopsies, the diagnostic accuracy approaches 100%. In Japan, the double-contrast air/barium study is used extensively for screening. Once diagnosis is made, CT is performed to evaluate local extension and to look for evidence of ascites or metastatic disease.

STAGING

Staging for stomach cancer is according to TNM (tumor, nodes, metastases) classification (Table 20-1).

TREATMENT

The theory behind curative resection involves en bloc primary tumor resection with wide disease-free margins

■ TABLE 20-1 American Joint Committee on Cancer (AJCC) TNM Classification of Carcinoma of the Stomach			
Primary Tumor (T)			
TX	Primary tumor cannot be assessed		
T0	No evidence of primary tumor		
Tis	Carcinoma in situ: intraepithelial tumor without invasion of the lamina propria		
T1	Tumor invades lamina propria or submucosa		
T2	Tumor invades muscularis propria or subserosa[†]		
T2a	Tumor invades muscularis propria		
T2b	Tumor invades subserosa		
T3	Tumor penetrates serosa (visceral peritoneum) without invasion of adjacent structures[‡]		
T4	Tumor invades adjacent structures[†]		
Regional Lymph Nodes (N)			
NX	Regional lymph node(s) cannot be assessed		
N0	No regional lymph node metastasis[§]		
N1	Metastasis in 1 to 6 regional lymph nodes		
N2	Metastasis in 7 to 15 regional lymph nodes		
N3	Metastasis in more than 15 regional lymph nodes		
Distant Metastasis (M)			
MX	Distant metastasis cannot be assessed		
M0	No distant metastasis		
M1	Distant metastasis		
Histologic Grade (G)			
Gx	Grade cannot be assessed		
G1	Well differentiated		
G2	Moderately differentiated		
G3	Poorly differentiated		
G4	Undifferentiated		
Stage Grouping			
Stage 0	Tis	N0	M0
Stage IA	T1	N0	M0
Stage IB	T1	N1	M0
	T2a/b	N0	M0
Stage II	T1	N2	M0
	T2a/b	N1	M0
	T3	N0	M0

(Continued)

TABLE 20-1 American Joint Committee on Cancer (AJCC) TNM Classification of Carcinoma of the Stomach *(continued)*			
Stage IIIA	T2a/b	N2	M0
	T3	N1	M0
	T4	N0	M0
Stage IIIB	T3	N2	M0
Stage IV	T4	N1-3	M0
	T1-3	N1-3	M0
	Any T	Any N	M1

†A tumor may penetrate the muscularis propria with extension into the gastrocolic or gastrohepatic ligaments, or into the greater or lesser omentum, without perforation of the visceral peritoneum covering these structures. In this case, the tumor is classified as T2. If there is perforation of the visceral peritoneum covering the gastric ligaments or the omentum, the tumor should be classified as T3.

‡The adjacent structures of the stomach include the spleen, transverse colon, liver, diaphragm, pancreas, abdominal wall, adrenal gland, kidney, small intestine, and retroperitoneum. Intramural extension to the duodenum or esophagus is classified by the depth of the greatest invasion in any of these sites, including the stomach.

§A designation of pN0 should be used if all examined lymph nodes are negative, regardless of the total number removed and examined.

Used with permission of the American Joint Committee on Cancer (AJCC), Chicago, Illinois. Original source: AJCC Cancer Staging Manual. 6th ed. New York, NY: Springer-Verlag; 2002.

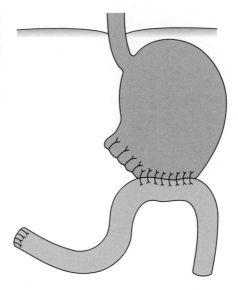

Figure 20-7 • Billroth II reconstruction after antral gastric cancer resection.

PROGNOSIS

The overall 5-year survival rate for gastric cancer in the United States is approximately 10%. Based on pathologic staging of tumors, the survival rate for stage I is 70%; stage II, 30%; stage III, 10%; and stage IV, 0%.

and disease-free lymph nodes. Tumors are located either in the proximal, middle, or distal stomach. The type of operation performed for cure depends on tumor location. Distal lesions located in the antral or prepyloric area are treated with subtotal gastrectomy and Billroth II or Roux-en-Y anastomosis (Fig. 20-7).

Midgastric and proximal lesions are treated with total gastrectomy, with extensive lymph node dissection. The lesser and greater omentum are removed, along with the spleen. If the body or tail of the pancreas is involved, distal pancreatectomy can be performed. Reconstruction is by Roux-en-Y anastomosis (Fig. 20-8).

Proximal lesions carry a poor prognosis, and surgical intervention is usually palliative. If there is extension into the distal esophagus, it is resected along with the cardia and lesser curvature. The remaining stomach tube is closed, and the proximal aspect is anastomosed to the midesophagus through a right thoracotomy. If extensive esophageal involvement is discovered, radical near-total gastrectomy and a near-complete esophagectomy are performed, with continuity restored using a distal transverse colon and proximal left colon interposition (Fig. 20-9).

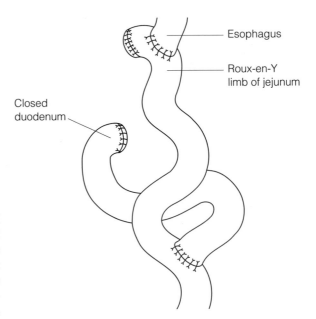

Esophagus

Roux-en-Y limb of jejunum

Closed duodenum

Figure 20-8 • Roux-en-Y esophagojejunostomy reconstruction after total gastrectomy.

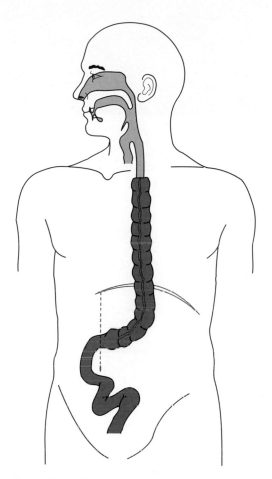

Figure 20-9 • Colonic interposition after near-total esophagectomy and near-total gastrectomy.

🔑 20-5 KEY POINTS

1. Benzopyrene, nitrosamines, and atrophic gastritis are thought to influence the development of gastric cancer.
2. Most tumors are located in the antral region and are either polypoid nodular, ulcerating, or superficial spreading tumors on gross inspection.
3. The pathologic staging of gastric cancer is based on the depth of invasion and lymph node status.
4. Tumor stage correlates closely with survival.
5. Signs of metastatic disease include Virchow node, Sister Joseph node, and Blumer shelf.
6. En bloc resection with Billroth II or Roux-en-Y anastomosis is usually performed when operating for gastric cancer.
7. Esophageal involvement requires esophagogastrectomy.

References

Gonzales RJ, Mansfield, PF. Adjuvant and neoadjuvant therapy for gastric cancer. *Surg Clin North Am.* 2005;85(5):1033–1051, viii.

Graham DY, Shiotani, A. Pathogenesis and therapy of gastric and duodenal ulcer disease. *Med Clin North Am.* 2002;86(6):1447–1466, viii.

Jansen EP. Optimal locoregional treatment in gastric cancer. *J Clin Oncol.* 2005;23(20):4509–4517.

Spleen

The spleen is a lymphatic organ located in the left upper abdominal quadrant. It contains the largest accumulation of lymphoid cells in the body. In addition to filtering the blood, it plays an important role in host defense. Splenic lymphocytes are involved in antigen recognition and plasma cell production, whereas splenic endothelial macrophages extract bacteria and damaged red blood cells from circulation by phagocytosis.

Surgical issues regarding the spleen are multiple and varied. Life-threatening hemorrhage from a lacerated spleen resulting from trauma is a common problem, requiring swift surgical intervention. Certain disease states, such as immune thrombocytopenic purpura (ITP) and the hemolytic anemias, are often treated by splenectomy when medical management fails. Splenectomy may be necessary as part of another operation, such as distal pancreatectomy. In addition, the traditional staging workup for Hodgkin disease has involved removal of the spleen to determine extent of disease, although this is now rarely performed.

ANATOMY

The spleen is embryologically derived from condensations of mesoderm in the dorsal mesogastrium of the developing gastrointestinal tract. In the mature abdomen, the spleen is found attached to the stomach by the gastrosplenic ligament and to the left kidney by the splenorenal ligament. Other supporting attachments include the splenocolic and splenophrenic ligaments (Fig. 21-1).

Accessory spleens are present in approximately 25% of patients. They are most often found in the splenic hilum and in the supporting splenic ligaments and greater omentum.

Arterial blood is mostly supplied via the splenic artery, which is one of three branches of the celiac axis (splenic, left gastric, common hepatic). At the hilum, the splenic artery divides into smaller branches that supply the several splenic segments. Additional arterial blood is supplied via the short gastric and left gastroepiploic vessels (Fig. 21-2).

Venous drainage is from segmental veins that join at the splenic hilum to form the splenic vein. Running behind the upper edge of the pancreas, the splenic vein joins with the superior mesenteric vein to form the portal vein.

🔑 21-1 KEY POINTS

1. The spleen is a lymphatic organ that plays roles in antigen recognition and blood filtering.
2. Possible indications for splenectomy include hemorrhage, disease states, surgical resections, and, rarely, staging for Hodgkin disease.
3. Accessory spleens occur in 25% of patients and are most commonly found in the splenic hilum.
4. Arterial blood is supplied via the splenic artery, the short gastric arteries, and branches of the left gastroepiploic artery.

SPLENIC HEMORRHAGE

The most common cause of splenic hemorrhage is blunt abdominal trauma. Nonpenetrating injury may cause disruption of the splenic capsule or frank laceration of the splenic parenchyma. Displaced rib fractures of the left lower chest often cause splenic laceration.

Splenic hemorrhage may also be iatrogenic. Intraoperative damage to the spleen may occur during unrelated abdominal surgery that results in bleeding controlled only by splenectomy. Estimates are that 20% of

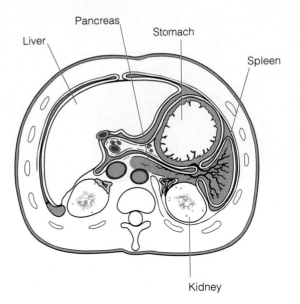

Figure 21-1 • Normal anatomic relations of the spleen.

splenectomies result from iatrogenic etiologies. Infectious diseases (mononucleosis, malaria) may damage the spleen to the point that unnoticed blunt trauma can cause "spontaneous" splenic rupture and hemorrhage.

HISTORY

Patients typically present with a recent history of trauma, usually to the left upper abdomen or left flank.

PHYSICAL EXAMINATION

Depending on the degree of splenic injury and hemoperitoneum, a physical examination may reveal left

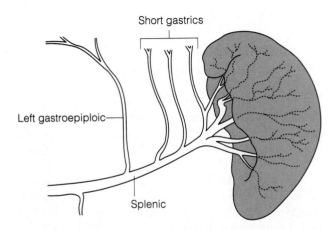

Figure 21-2 • Arterial supply of the spleen.

upper quadrant abdominal tenderness, left lower rib fractures, abdominal distention, peritonitis, and hypovolemic shock.

DIAGNOSTIC EVALUATION

Computed tomographic (CT) scan, abdominal ultrasound, and peritoneal lavage can be used to detect intraperitoneal blood. In hemodynamically stable patients, CT can demonstrate the degree of both splenic injury and hemoperitoneum.

TREATMENT

For patients with splenic injury who are hemodynamically stable and without evidence of ongoing hemorrhage, nonoperative management with close hemodynamic monitoring has become the accepted treatment of choice. In children, nonoperative management is widely applied, due to the increased incidence of overwhelming postsplenectomy sepsis (OPSS) seen in the pediatric population. For patients with known or suspected splenic injury who are hemodynamically unstable, operative intervention is indicated to control ongoing hemorrhage.

Once in the operating room, the decision to perform splenic repair (splenorrhaphy) versus splenectomy is based on the degree of injury to the parenchyma and blood supply of the organ. Relatively minor injuries, such as a small capsular laceration with minor oozing, may be repaired, whereas a fragmented spleen with involvement of the hilar vessels necessitates surgical removal.

🔑 21-2 KEY POINTS

1. Hemorrhage secondary to trauma is the most common indication for splenectomy.
2. Nonoperative management or organ-sparing splenorrhaphy can be attempted to avoid the risk of overwhelming postsplenectomy sepsis, especially in children.
3. Hemodynamically stable patients can be managed nonoperatively.

IMMUNE THROMBOCYTOPENIC PURPURA

ITP is an autoimmune hematologic disease in which antiplatelet immunoglobulin G (IgG) antibodies, produced largely in the spleen, are directed against a platelet-associated antigen, resulting in platelet destruction by the reticuloendothelial system and subsequent thrombocytopenia. The disease is typically seen in young women, who may present with complaints of menorrhagia, easy bruising, mucosal bleeding, and petechiae. Men may present with complaints of prolonged bleeding after shaving trauma.

TREATMENT

Initial therapy is with corticosteroids, which improve platelet counts after 3 to 7 days of therapy. For prolonged active bleeding, platelet transfusions should be administered to achieve hemostasis.

Few patients enjoy complete and sustained remission with steroid treatment alone. Patients typically become refractory to medical treatment, and thrombocytopenia recurs. Splenectomy is then indicated. Patients should receive immunization with the pneumococcal polyvalent polysaccharide (Pneumovax), *Haemophilus influenzae*, and *Neisseria meningitidis* meningococcus vaccines, preferably at least 2 weeks before surgery. After splenectomy, normal platelet counts develop in approximately 80% of patients because the organ of both significant antiplatelet antibody production and platelet destruction is removed.

HYPERSPLENISM

Hypersplenism describes a state of increased splenic function that results in various hematologic abnormalities, which can be normalized by splenectomy. Elevated splenic function causes a depression of the formed blood elements, leading to a compensatory hyperplasia of the bone marrow.

HISTORY

As in ITP, most patients are women who present with signs of anemia, recurrent infections, or easy bruising.

PHYSICAL EXAMINATION

Abdominal examination reveals splenomegaly.

DIAGNOSTIC EVALUATION

Peripheral blood smear may reveal leukopenia, anemia, thrombocytopenia, or pancytopenia. Bone marrow biopsy shows pancellular hyperplasia.

TREATMENT

Splenectomy may produce hematologic improvement.

HEMOLYTIC ANEMIAS

Hemolytic anemias are characterized by an elevated rate of red cell destruction from either a congenital or acquired etiology. Congenital hemolytic anemias result from basic defects of the cell membrane (hereditary spherocytosis), hemoglobin synthesis (thalassemia), hemoglobin structure (sickle cell anemia), or cellular metabolism (glucose-6-phosphate dehydrogenase [G-6-PD] deficiency). Acquired autoimmune hemolytic anemias result when antibodies are produced that are directed against the body's own red blood cells.

DIAGNOSTIC EVALUATION

A positive direct Coombs test demonstrates complexed antibodies on the red blood cell membrane. Warm-reactive antibodies are IgG, and cold-reactive antibodies are immunoglobulin M (IgM).

TREATMENT

The role of splenectomy in treating hemolytic anemias depends on the particular disease process. For example, red blood cell survival normalizes after splenectomy for hereditary spherocytosis, whereas operative intervention has no role in the treatment of anemia of G-6-PD deficiency that is secondary to a defect of metabolism, not cellular structure. Occasionally, splenectomy may be useful in selected patients with sickle cell anemia and thalassemia. Patients with autoimmune hemolytic anemias undergo initial steroid treatment and progress to splenectomy only after medical treatment failure.

HODGKIN DISEASE STAGING

Because of a greater reliance on CT scans and the favorable success of salvage chemotherapy in the treatment of Hodgkin lymphoma, the need for determining whether disease is present across the diaphragm by means of laparotomy and splenectomy has sharply declined. Treatment with salvage chemotherapy after local radiation failure still carries a highly favorable outcome in most cases. Therefore, splenectomy for staging Hodgkin disease is now rarely performed.

OVERWHELMING POSTSPLENECTOMY SEPSIS

Asplenic individuals are at greater risk for developing fulminant bacteremia because of decreased opsonic activity, decreased levels of IgM, and decreased clearance of bacteria from the blood after splenectomy. As a rule, children are at greater risk for development of sepsis than are adults, and fatal sepsis is more common after splenectomy for hematologic disorders than after trauma. The risk of sepsis is higher in the first postoperative year, and, for adults, each subsequent year carries approximately a 1% chance of developing sepsis. The clinical picture of OPSS is the onset of high fever followed by circulatory collapse from septic shock. Disseminated intravascular coagulation often occurs. The offending pathogens are the encapsulated bacteria *Streptococcus pneumoniae*, *H. influenzae*, and *N. meningitidis*.

Concern regarding OPSS has spurred efforts to perform partial splenectomy or splenorrhaphy in trauma to preserve splenic function. Vaccination against pneumococcal sepsis with Pneumovax, *H. influenzae*, and *N. meningitidis* should be administered to all surgically and functionally asplenic patients.

✎ 21-3 KEY POINTS

1. Immune thrombocytopenic purpura, hypersplenism, and specific hemolytic anemias are disease states for which splenectomy may be indicated.
2. Splenectomy for staging Hodgkin disease is now rarely performed, because of improved imaging modalities (computed tomography scan) and the success of chemotherapy.
3. The risk of overwhelming postsplenectomy sepsis (OPSS) is greater in children than in adults. High fever and septic shock are often accompanied by disseminated intravascular coagulation.
4. *Streptococcus pneumoniae, Haemophilus influenzae,* and *Neisseria meningitidis* are encapsulated organisms that are responsible for causing OPSS.
5. Vaccination against *S. pneumoniae, H. influenzae,* and *N. meningitidis* should be administered to all surgically and functionally asplenic patients.

References

Cines DB, McMillan R. Management of adult idiopathic thrombocytopenic purpura. *Annu Rev Med.* 2006;56:425–442.

Davidson RN, Wall RA. Prevention and management of infections in patients without a spleen. *Clin Microbiol Infect.* 2001;7(21):657–660.

Velmahos GC, et al. Nonoperative treatment of blunt injury to solid abdominal organs: a prospective study. *Arch Surg.* 2003;138(8):844–851.

Thyroid Gland

Surgical thyroid disease encompasses those conditions in which partial or complete removal of the thyroid gland is required due to goiter and hyperthyroid conditions that are unresponsive to medical management or due to benign and malignant neoplastic disease.

ANATOMY AND PHYSIOLOGY

The thyroid gland is derived embryologically from an evagination of the floor of the pharynx at the base of the tongue. The developing thyroid descends along a midline course via the thyroglossal duct to its final position as a bilobed gland overlying the lower half of the thyroid cartilage. The two lateral lobes of the fully developed gland are connected by a median isthmus. In 75% of individuals, the distal thyroglossal remnant extends superiorly from the isthmus and is called the *pyramidal lobe*. Arterial blood is supplied via the paired superior and inferior thyroid arteries, and venous drainage is via the paired superior, middle, and inferior thyroid veins (Fig. 22-1).

Of key importance to the surgeon is anatomic knowledge of the recurrent laryngeal nerve (Fig. 22-2). Bilateral vagus nerves descend from the neck into the chest. The right vagus branches into the right recurrent laryngeal nerve, which loops under the right subclavian artery from anterior to posterior and ascends superiorly in the right tracheoesophageal groove. In 5% of patients, the right laryngeal nerve may be nonrecurrent, taking a more direct course into the larynx. The left vagus branches into the left recurrent laryngeal nerve, which loops in a similar anterior-to-posterior fashion around the arch of the aorta and ascends along the left tracheoesophageal groove. The recurrent laryngeal nerves travel posteromedial to their respective thyroid lobes and enter the larynx via the cricothyroid membrane to innervate the abductor

muscles of the true vocal cords. Injury during thyroidectomy results in ipsilateral vocal cord paralysis and subsequent hoarseness.

As a result of aberrant migration of the developing thyroid gland, several anatomic variances can be seen (Fig. 22-3). Complete failure of migration from the base of the tongue results in a lingual thyroid. The entire mass of thyroid tissue is located in the posterior tongue, and airway obstruction may result if goiter develops. Incomplete migration can result in thyroid tissue being found anywhere between the base of the tongue and the root of the neck. Lastly, thyroid tissue may migrate beyond the level of the thyroid cartilage into the substernal region, where occasionally a substernal goiter develops.

Persistence of the thyroglossal duct results in a thyroglossal cyst or fistula. Thyroglossal cysts are most commonly seen in children and appear as a single painless lump in the midline that moves with swallowing. Surgical excision of the cyst is corrective. Thyroglossal duct fistulae appear as midline sinus tracts. Because the fistula is an embryologic remnant, it ascends superiorly through the middle of the hyoid bone, often to its origin at the base of the tongue. Surgical excision of the fistula requires resection of the middle portion of the hyoid bone.

The thyroid gland determines the metabolic pace of the body. Increased levels of thyroid hormone and loss of the normal negative feedback mechanism result in hyperthyroidism. The main etiologies of hyperthyroidism are (a) diffuse toxic goiter (Graves disease), (b) toxic multinodular goiter (Plummer disease), and (c) toxic adenoma. Surgical treatment of these disorders involves either excision of localized diseased tissue, as in the case of adenoma, or complete excision of the majority of the gland, as in Graves or toxic multinodular goiter.

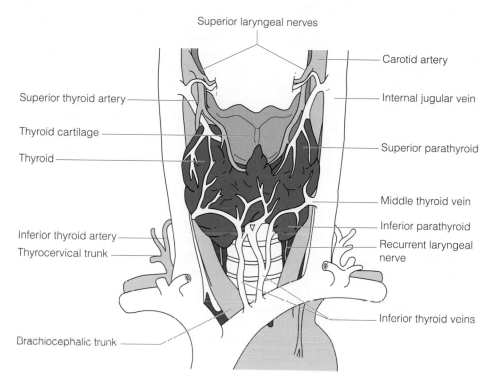

Figure 22-1 • Anatomy of the thyroid gland.

GRAVES DISEASE

The most common cause of hyperthyroidism in the United States and Europe is Graves disease. This autoimmune disorder is caused by thyroid-stimulating immunoglobulins that target the thyroid-stimulating hormone (TSH) receptor of the thyroid gland. The hyperstimulated gland releases excessive amounts of hormone, resulting in the classic clinical picture of goiter: exophthalmos, pretibial myxedema, and the signs and

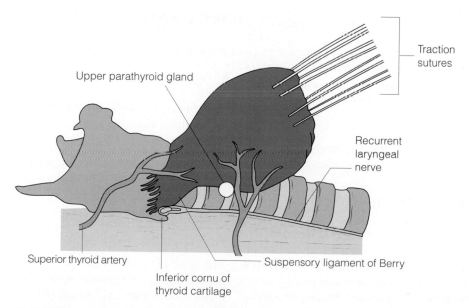

Figure 22-2 • Course of the recurrent laryngeal nerve.

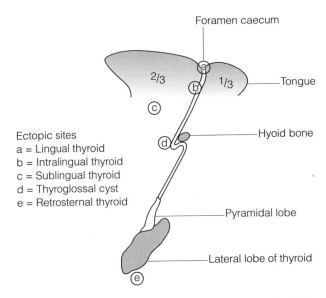

Foramen caecum

2/3   1/3 — Tongue

— Hyoid bone

Ectopic sites
a = Lingual thyroid
b = Intralingual thyroid
c = Sublingual thyroid
d = Thyroglossal cyst
e = Retrosternal thyroid

— Pyramidal lobe

— Lateral lobe of thyroid

Figure 22-3 • Migration of the thyroid via the thyroglossal duct and possible ectopic sites of development and duct remnants.

symptoms of hyperthyroidism. The exact pathogenesis remains unclear; however, evidence of a genetic component exists in many cases. Families with Graves disease exhibit an overall increased incidence of thyroid disorders and increased levels of circulating antithyroid antibodies. Individuals and families with Graves disease also have higher incidences of other autoimmune disorders, such as insulin-dependent diabetes mellitus, rheumatoid arthritis, and Addison disease.

HISTORY

The typical presentation of hyperthyroidism involves complaints of unexplained nervousness and sweating, heat intolerance, weight loss, palpitations, an enlarging neck mass, and ocular prominence. As patients present at different stages of disease, the subtle findings of early disease differ dramatically from the florid exophthalmos, dyspnea, and agitation of more advanced cases.

PHYSICAL EXAMINATION

Patients are usually agitated, irritable, or nervous. The enlarged gland is palpable and often visibly apparent. Due to increased vascularity, a thrill may be felt or a bruit auscultated over the enlarged lobes.

The most notable and dramatic finding is exophthalmos, caused by edema of the retrobulbar fat pad, forcing the globe anteriorly. Increased sympathetic tone

secondary to excess thyroid hormone causes eyelid retraction, leading to the pronounced Graves "stare."

Skin examination reveals myxedema, a raised plaque-like skin change seen typically in a pretibial distribution. Cardiac examination demonstrates sinus tachycardia, hyperdynamism, systolic flow murmurs, and occasionally atrial fibrillation.

DIAGNOSTIC EVALUATION

Thyroid function tests yield the information necessary for diagnosing Graves disease. T3 and T4 levels are elevated, due to gland hyperstimulation, and the TSH level is low, due to the negative feedback exerted by circulating thyroid hormones. If T3 and T4 levels are within normal limits, radioactive iodine uptake testing will show increased uptake secondary to increased glandular activity.

Thyrotropin-releasing hormone (TRH) testing shows a negative response in Graves disease. TSH does not rise in response to intravenous infusion of TRH, because pituitary secretion has been inhibited by negative feedback.

DIFFERENTIAL DIAGNOSIS

In addition to hyperthyroidism, one should consider thyroiditis, factitious hyperthyroidism, and anxiety disorder as possible diagnoses.

TREATMENT

Hyperthyroidism of Graves disease is treated by

- Antithyroid medication to reduce glandular hormone secretion,
- Radioiodine ablation to reduce the functional glandular mass, or
- Surgical excision.

The appropriate treatment choice is determined by such considerations as pregnancy status, surgical risk, and treatment side effects.

Antithyroid Medication

The goal of antithyroid medication is to return the patient to a euthyroid state. Two thiocarbamide medications—propylthiouracil (PTU) and methimazole (Tapazole)—inhibit thyroid hormone synthesis. In addition, PTU inhibits peripheral conversion of T4 to T3.

Despite the ability of antithyroid medications to control the signs and symptoms of hyperthyroidism, there is a high recurrence rate. Hence, such medications are used for long-term treatment of patients who are expected to undergo remission as indicated by mild laboratory abnormalities and a small goiter.

Adjunctive drug therapy includes beta-blockers to control the signs and symptoms of thyrotoxicosis. Propranolol is used to dampen the increased sympathetic tone brought on by circulating thyroid hormones. Iodide is used to inhibit thyroid hormone release directly and to rapidly treat patients with severe disease. Potassium iodide (Lugol solution) can also be used preoperatively before elective thyroidectomy to reduce glandular vascularity.

Radioactive Iodine Therapy

Radioactive ablation of the thyroid with iodine-131 is simple and effective. The goal of therapy is to reduce the functional mass of thyroid tissue to achieve a euthyroid level of secretion. However, the final result is often complete glandular ablation, with subsequent permanent hypothyroidism, requiring lifelong thyroid hormone replacement. Radioactive iodine therapy is useful for most patients, except pregnant women and newborns.

Subtotal Thyroidectomy

Surgical intervention is appropriate for patients with contraindications to radioactive iodine therapy and for those who are unable to tolerate or are unresponsive to antithyroid medications. Children and young adults are the majority of such patients. As with radioiodine therapy, the goal of surgical treatment is to reduce the mass of thyroid tissue to a level at which euthyroid levels of hormone are secreted by residual tissue. Despite the low operative risk of the procedure, significant complications can include recurrent laryngeal nerve injury with vocal cord paralysis, permanent hypothyroidism, and surgical hypoparathyroidism. Despite undergoing surgery, recurrent hyperthyroidism occurs in approximately 5% of patients.

The operation is performed through a curvilinear necklace incision, extending to the sternocleidomastoid muscles bilaterally. Of key importance is to avoid injury to the recurrent laryngeal nerves, parathyroid glands, and external branches of the superior laryngeal nerves.

FOLLOW-UP

After treatment, thyroid function tests should be used to ensure that the patient is euthyroid. This is important, because up to 50% of patients may develop postoperative hypothyroidism and require thyroid hormone replacement therapy.

THYROID CANCER

Thyroid cancers are relatively uncommon—they account for only approximately 1% of all malignancies. The four thyroid cancer types are papillary, follicular, medullary, and anaplastic. The tumor types differ in histologic appearance, malignant behavior, and treatment response. Indolent papillary cancer carries a favorable 80% 10-year survival rate, whereas undifferentiated anaplastic cancer is invariably fatal. Anaplastic thyroid cancer is one of the most lethal cancers known, with an average life expectancy of 5 months from the time of diagnosis. Follicular and medullary cancers occupy the middle ground. Depending on the tumor type, surgical therapy has variable success.

PATHOGENESIS

Although the etiology of most thyroid cancer is unknown, cancer of the thyroid has been experimentally induced by exposure to radiation, goitrogenic medications, and iodide deficiency. Knowledge of radiation-induced carcinogenesis evolved from experience with the use of external-beam radiation as medical therapy in the twentieth century. It was noted that thyroid cancer, usually of the papillary type, subsequently developed in a significant number of children irradiated for the treatment of acne, enlarged tonsils, or hemangiomas. A direct dose-response relationship was identified, showing that the incidence of malignancy was proportional to the radiation dose received. Eventually it was discovered that ionizing radiation exerts a dual carcinogenic role: the disruption of cellular deoxyribonucleic acid (DNA) and the inducement of chronic TSH stimulation of the thyroid gland by damaging the capacity to produce thyroid hormone, which is necessary for negative feedback.

HISTORY

Patients usually present for surgical evaluation after an asymptomatic painless thyroid nodule is discovered on routine physical examination. A systemic workup for a newly diagnosed thyroid nodule is necessary to determine the biologic nature of the nodule and to rule out cancer. Important historic information includes the duration of nodule existence, rate of enlargement, presence of voice changes, dysphagia, prior radiation exposure from medical or military sources, radioiodine therapy in childhood, family history of medullary cancer, and history of iodide deficiency suggested by residence in a geographic area of endemic goiter.

PHYSICAL EXAMINATION

Physical findings may range from a single discrete nodule in a single lobe to large bulky disease with evidence of distant metastasis. In general, carcinomas are nontender on palpation; however, pain may arise after hemorrhage into a necrotic tumor or by compression of local structures. Hoarseness is often a sign of malignancy, indicating involvement of the recurrent laryngeal nerve. An enlarging fixed nodule with associated adenopathy and symptoms of dysphagia also suggest malignancy.

DIFFERENTIAL DIAGNOSIS

The differential diagnosis of a thyroid nodule includes follicular adenoma, multinodular goiter, colloid nodule, Hashimoto thyroiditis, thyroid cyst, thyroid lymphoma, papillary thyroid cancer, follicular thyroid cancer, medullary thyroid cancer, anaplastic thyroid cancer, metastatic cancer, and parathyroid mass.

DIAGNOSTIC EVALUATION

Standard thyroid function tests reveal the functional status of the gland; results are rarely abnormal in patients with thyroid cancer. The single most important diagnostic study is percutaneous fine-needle aspiration (FNA), because it provides a tissue diagnosis. Other studies include radionuclide thyroid scanning, which only demonstrates the functional status of a nodule by showing whether a nodule is "hot" or "cold." A hot functioning nodule takes up high levels of radioactive iodide tracer, and a cold nodule indicates low uptake and minimal function. Overall, the majority of hot nodules are benign, and approximately 5% of cold nodules are malignant. Thyroid ultrasound is used to determine whether a nodule is solid or cystic, to assess nodule size, or to identify impalpable nodules. Solid nodules are more likely to be cancerous

than are cystic lesions. For patients suspected of having medullary cancer based on family history, serum calcitonin levels should be checked after a calcium-pentagastrin infusion test. An elevated calcitonin level defines a positive result and obviates the need for FNA.

STAGING

Staging for thyroid cancer is according to TNM classification (Table 22-1).

TREATMENT

Papillary

Usually associated with exposure to ionizing radiation, papillary thyroid cancer is often multicentric and bilateral, spreading slowly via lymphatic channels to lymph nodes and by direct extension into surrounding structures. Only 5% of patients with papillary cancer present with distant metastases. For tumors <1.5 cm and for disease clinically confined to one lobe with no extracapsular extension, thyroid lobectomy is usually performed. Due to the multicentric and often bilateral nature of the disease, however, some surgeons advocate total thyroidectomy, because a more extensive operation is associated with lower rates of recurrence and better long-term survival.

Follicular

Found more commonly in iodide-deficient regions, follicular thyroid cancer usually manifests as a solitary thyroid mass. FNA cytology is unable to distinguish follicular adenoma from carcinoma, as angioinvasion and capsular invasion can only be seen histologically. Tumors invade vascular structures, and metastasis is by hematologic spread to brain, bone, lungs, and liver. Total thyroidectomy is indicated, and radioactive iodine ablation is usually performed postoperatively.

Medullary

Typically seen as part of multiple endocrine neoplasia disease, heritable medullary thyroid cancer is usually multicentric and bilateral, with early metastasis to cervical lymph nodes. Sporadic cases make up the majority of medullary cancers. Total thyroidectomy is performed, with additional neck dissection if lymph node metastases are present.

TABLE 22-1 American Joint Committee on Cancer (AJCC) TNM Classification of Thyroid Carcinoma

Primary Tumor (T)

Note: All categories may be subdivided: (a) solitary tumor, (b) multifocal tumor (the largest determines the classification).

TX	Primary tumor cannot be assessed
T0	No evidence of primary tumor
T1	Tumor 2 cm or less in greatest dimension limited to the thyroid
T2	Tumor more than 2 cm but not more than 4 cm in greatest dimension limited to the thyroid
T3	Tumor more than 4 cm in greatest dimension limited to the thyroid or any tumor with minimal extrathyroid extension (e.g., extension to sternothyroid muscle or perithyroid soft tissues)
T4a	Tumor of any size extending beyond the thyroid capsule to invade subcutaneous soft tissues, larynx, trachea, esophagus, or recurrent laryngeal nerve
T4b	Tumor invades prevertebral fascia or encases carotid artery or mediastinal vessels

All anaplastic carcinomas are considered T4 tumors.

T4a	Intrathyroidal anaplastic carcinoma—surgically resectable
T4b	Extrathyroidal anaplastic carcinoma—surgically unresectable

Regional Lymph Nodes (N)

Regional lymph nodes are the central compartment, lateral cervical, and upper mediastinal lymph nodes.

NX	Regional lymph node(s) cannot be assessed
N0	No regional lymph node metastasis
N1	Regional lymph nodes metastasis
N1a	Metastasis to Level VI (pretracheal, paratracheal, and prelaryngeal/Delphian lymph nodes)
N1b	Metastasis to unilateral, bilateral, or contralateral cervical or superior mediastinal lymph nodes

Distant Metastasis (M)

MX	Distant metastasis cannot be assessed
M0	No distant metastasis
M1	Distant metastasis

Stage Grouping:

Separate stage groupings are recommended for follicular, medullary, and anaplastic (undifferentiated) carcinoma.

Papillary or Follicular

Under 45 years

Stage I	Any T	Any N	M0
Stage II	Any T	Any N	M1

Papillary or Follicular

45 years and older

Stage I	T1	N0	M0
Stage II	T2	N0	M0
Stage III	T3	N0	M0
	T1	N1a	M0
	T2	N1a	M0
	T3	N1a	M0
Stage IVA	T4a	N0	M0
	T4a	N1a	M0
	T1	N1b	M0
	T2	N1b	M0
	T3	N1b	M0
	T4a	N1b	M0
Stage IVB	T4b	Any N	M0
Stage IVC	Any T	Any N	M1

Medullary carcinoma

Stage I	T1	N0	M0
Stage II	T2	N0	M0
Stage III	T3	N0	M0
	T1	N1a	M0
	T2	N1a	M0
	T3	N1a	M0
Stage IVA	T4a	N0	M0
	T4a	N1a	M0
	T1	N1b	M0
	T2	N1b	M0
	T3	N1b	M0
	T4a	N1b	M0
Stage IVB	T4b	Any N	M0
Stage IVC	Any T	Any N	M1

Anaplastic carcinoma

All anaplastic carcinomas are considered Stage IV.

(Continued)

■ TABLE 22-1 American Joint Committee on Cancer (AJCC) TNM Classification of Thyroid Carcinoma *(continued)*

Stage IVA	T4a	Any N	M0
Stage IVB	T4b	Any N	M0
Stage IVC	Any T	Any N	M1

Histopathologic Type

There are four major histopathologic types:

- Papillary carcinoma (including follicular variant of papillary carcinoma)
- Follicular carcinoma (including Hurthle cell carcinoma)
- Medullary carcinoma
- Undifferentiated (anaplastic) carcinoma

Stage 0	Tis	N0	M0
Stage IA	T1	N0	M0
Stage IB	T1	N1	M0
	T2a/b	N0	M0
Stage II	T1	N2	M0
	T2a/b	N1	M0
	T3	N0	M0
Stage IIIA	T2a/b	N2	M0
	T3	N1	M0
	T4	N0	M0
Stage IIIB	T3	N2	M0
Stage IV	T4	N1-3	M0
	T1-3	N1-3	M0
	Any T	Any N	M1

Used with permission of the American Joint Committee on Cancer (AJCC), Chicago, Illinois. Original source: AJCC Cancer Staging Manual. 6th ed. New York, NY: Springer-Verlag; 2002.

🔑 22-1 KEY POINTS

1. The thyroid gland is derived from an evagination at the base of the tongue, followed by migration into the neck via the thyroglossal duct. Failure of thyroid migration results in a lingual thyroid, whereas persistence of the thyroglossal duct results in a thyroglossal cyst or fistula.
2. The recurrent laryngeal nerve may be damaged during surgery, causing ipsilateral vocal cord paralysis and hoarseness.
3. Graves disease, toxic multinodular goiter, and toxic adenoma are the main etiologies of hyperthyroidism.
4. Graves disease is an autoimmune disorder caused by thyroid-stimulating immunoglobulins that target thyroid-stimulating hormone (TSH) receptors of the thyroid gland.
5. T3 and T4 levels are elevated in Graves disease, whereas the TSH level is low due to negative feedback.
6. Management of Graves disease includes antithyroid medications, radioiodine ablation, or surgical excision.
7. Complications of subtotal thyroidectomy include recurrent laryngeal nerve injury, permanent hypothyroidism, and surgical hypoparathyroidism.
8. The four types of thyroid cancer, in order of increasing malignancy, are papillary, follicular, medullary, and anaplastic.
9. Fine-needle aspiration is the most important diagnostic study for evaluation of a thyroid nodule.
10. Patients with hereditary medullary cancer have an elevated calcitonin level on calcium-pentagastrin testing.

Anaplastic

Lethal cancers seen more frequently in regions with endemic goiter, anaplastic thyroid cancers usually present as rapidly enlarging neck masses. Extremely aggressive tumor invasion into vital neck structures may cause dysphagia and dyspnea. Tracheal invasion is common, and tracheostomy may be required to maintain airway patency. Such invasiveness usually precludes surgical resection, and attempts at palliation with radiation therapy and chemotherapy have limited success.

References

Lado-Abeal J, Weiss RE. Thyroid nodules: diagnosis and therapy. *Curr Opin Oncol*. 2002;14(1):46–52.

Schulumberger MJ. Medical progress: papillary and follicular thyroid carcinoma. *N Engl J Med*. 1998;338:297–306.

Weetman AP. Medical progress: Graves' disease. *N Engl J Med*. 2000;343:1236–1248.

23 Trauma

Traumatic injury and death are a major problem in the United States, where approximately 60 million injuries occur annually. Trauma is the leading cause of death in the first four decades of life and the third leading cause of death overall, trailing only cancer and coronary artery disease. Although approximately 150,000 traumatic deaths occur annually, the rate of disability from trauma is three times greater than mortality. Therefore, issues relating to trauma care are of importance to all medical and surgical specialists, from the trauma surgeon to the rehabilitation specialist.

Death due to trauma has been shown to occur in a trimodal distribution, during three identifiable time periods. The first peak of death occurs within seconds to minutes of injury. Lethal injury to the body's vital anatomic structures leads to rapid death, unless immediate advanced intervention is performed. The second peak of death occurs within minutes to several hours after the injury. Death during this second period is usually due to progressive neurologic, cardiovascular, or pulmonary compromise. It is during this intermediate period that patients have the greatest chance of salvage and toward which organized trauma care is focused. Rapid resuscitation, coupled with the identification and treatment of potentially lethal injuries, is the goal. The final third peak of death occurs several days to weeks after initial injury, usually secondary to sepsis and multiorgan system failure.

This chapter discusses trauma management during the aforementioned second period. Specifically, the steps of the initial assessment performed when the trauma patient arrives at the hospital emergency room, the primary survey of the patient (ABCs), resuscitation, the secondary survey (head to toe), and the institution of definitive care are examined.

PRIMARY SURVEY

The focus of the primary survey is to identify immediately life-threatening conditions and to prevent death. Without a patent airway, adequate gas exchange, or sufficient intravascular volume, any patient will die. Therefore, a simple mnemonic—ABCDE—is used to direct the primary survey:

Airway with cervical spine control
Breathing and ventilation
Circulation and hemorrhage control
Disability and neurologic assessment
Exposure to enable examination

(A)

The airway is immediately inspected to ensure that patency and any causes of airway obstruction are identified (foreign body, facial fracture, tracheal/laryngeal disruption, cervical spine injury). Cervical spine control must be maintained at all times—patients with multitrauma must be assumed to have cervical spine injury until cleared radiographically. The chin thrust and jaw lift are methods of initially establishing airway patency while simultaneously protecting the cervical spine.

(B)

Once airway patency is established, the patient's ability to breathe must be assessed. Normal function of the lungs, chest wall, and diaphragm is necessary for ventilation and gas exchange to occur. Auscultation, visual inspection, and palpation of the chest may indicate the presence of a tension pneumothorax, open pneumothorax, massive hemothorax, or flail chest segment with underlying pulmonary contusion. Needle decompression, chest tube placement, or endotracheal intubation may be required to ensure adequate ventilation.

(C)

Hypotension secondary to hemorrhage can result from both penetrating and blunt trauma. External hemorrhage can usually be identified and controlled by direct manual pressure. Tourniquets should be avoided, because they cause distal ischemia. Internal hemorrhage is more difficult to identify. Therefore, hypotension without signs of external hemorrhage must be assumed to be due to intra-abdominal or intrathoracic injury or from fractures of the pelvis or long bones. The hypovolemic hypotensive patient usually exhibits a diminished level of consciousness as cerebral blood flow is reduced, the pulse is rapid and thready, and the skin is pale and clammy.

(D)

Traumatic injuries may cause damage to the central and peripheral nervous systems. Spinal cord injuries are most commonly seen in the cervical and lumbar regions. The thoracic spine is less prone to injury due to the rigidity of the bony thorax. Complete spinal cord injury affects all neurologic function below a specific level of the cord. Incomplete spinal cord injury exhibits sacral sparing and may involve (a) the central portion of the cord, as in the central cord syndrome; (b) a single side of the cord, as in Brown-Séquard syndrome; or (c) the anterior portion of the cord, as in anterior cord syndrome. A rapid assessment of disability and neurologic function is vital so that drug therapy and physical maneuvers can be initiated to prevent further neurologic injury.

(E)

Exposure of the trauma patient is important for the entire body to be examined and injuries diagnosed. Complete exposure entails removing all clothing from the patient so a thorough examination can be performed, allowing for identification of entry and exit wounds, extremity deformities, contusions, or lacerations.

RESUSCITATION

The resuscitation phase of trauma management occurs almost simultaneously with the initial survey: Once a life-threatening condition is identified, the appropriate management is initiated. Airway control and ventilation are the first priorities for any trauma patient.

Airway control in the conscious patient can be achieved with an easily inserted nasopharyngeal trumpet; an oropharyngeal airway is used in the unconscious patient. Definitive control of the airway and enhanced ability to ventilate and oxygenate the patient are achieved with endotracheal intubation. Tube placement may be via the nasal or oral route. Nasotracheal intubation is a useful technique for patients with cervical spine injuries; however, it is contraindicated when midface or basilar skull fractures are suspected. When the trachea cannot be intubated, a surgical airway is indicated. Jet insufflation of the airway after needle cricothyroidotomy can adequately oxygenate patients for 30 to 45 minutes. Surgical cricothyroidotomy with the insertion of a tracheostomy or endotracheal tube allows prolonged ventilation and oxygenation.

Injuries to the chest may acutely impair the ability to provide adequate ventilation. The chest must be examined for evidence of tension pneumothorax, open pneumothorax, hemothorax, and flail chest. The clinical picture of hypotension, tachycardia, tracheal deviation, neck vein distention, and diminished unilateral breath sounds suggests the diagnosis of tension pneumothorax. Immediate decompression by inserting a needle catheter into the second intercostal space in the midclavicular line is indicated, followed by definitive treatment with chest tube insertion into the fifth intercostal space at the anterior axillary line just lateral to the nipple. Open pneumothorax requires closure of the chest wall defect. Hemothorax necessitates the insertion of a large-caliber chest tube for drainage of blood. Most patients with flail chest secondary to multiple rib fractures have underlying pulmonary contusion and may require eventual intubation to prevent hypoxia.

Hemorrhage leading to hypovolemic shock is the most common cause of postinjury death in the trauma patient. Rapid fluid resuscitation and hemorrhage control are the keys to restoring adequate circulating blood volume. The fluid status of patients can be quickly evaluated by assessing their hemodynamics (hypotension and tachycardia), their level of consciousness (adequacy of cerebral perfusion), the color of their skin (pale skin indicates significant exsanguination), and the presence and character of the pulse (absent central pulses indicate profound hypovolemic shock). All sources of external hemorrhage must be identified and treated by applying direct pressure. Indiscriminate hemostat usage should be avoided, because it may crush and damage surrounding neurovascular structures. Sources of internal hemorrhage are usually hidden and are suspected by unstable hemodynamics. Internal bleeding may occur in the thorax as a result of cardiovascular or pulmonary injury, in the abdomen from splenic or liver lacerations, or into the soft tissues surrounding femur or pelvic fractures.

Fluid resuscitation of the hypovolemic hypotensive patient requires establishing adequate intravenous access. Two large-bore intravenous catheters (14 gauge) should be placed in upper extremity veins and rapid infusion of a balanced salt solution (lactated Ringer or normal saline) initiated. If the pattern of injury allows, central access via the femoral vein approach using larger-diameter catheters maximizes the rate of fluid administration. If percutaneous access is unsuccessful, a cutdown of the greater saphenous vein at the antero-medial ankle is required. After intravenous access is established, bolus infusion of crystalloid solution should be replaced with O negative or type-specific blood once it becomes available.

TRAUMA RADIOGRAPHS

For patients with blunt trauma (automobile crashes, falls), three standard radiographic studies are required to assess the neck, chest, and pelvis: cross-table lateral cervical spine, anteroposterior chest, and anteroposte-rior pelvis. Obtaining these three x-rays early in the resuscitation process allows potentially neurologically disabling cervical spine injuries, life-threatening chest wall and cardiopulmonary injuries, and pelvic injuries to be identified and immediately treated. For patients with penetrating trauma (gunshot, stabbing, impal-ing), an anteroposterior chest film and other films per-taining to the site of injury should be obtained.

SECONDARY SURVEY

The secondary survey begins after the airway, breath-ing, and circulation have been assessed and resuscita-tion has been initiated. This secondary survey is a head-to-toe evaluation of the body, during which additional areas of injury are identified. A meticulous examina-tion during this phase of the trauma evaluation mini-mizes the chance of missing an important finding.

The final phase of acute trauma care is instituting definitive treatment. This may entail simple wound care in the emergency room for minor injuries or, if the injuries warrant, transportation to the operating room for surgical treatment.

23-1 KEY POINTS

1. Trauma is the leading cause of death in the first four decades of life.
2. Trauma is the third leading cause of death overall, after cancer and heart disease.
3. Traumatic death occurs in a trimodal distribution.
4. Trauma care involves the primary survey, resuscita-tion, secondary survey, and definitive care.
5. The primary survey identifies immediately life-threatening injuries involving the airway, breath-ing, and circulation.
6. Resuscitation involves airway control and ventila-tion and fluid infusion after intravenous access is obtained.
7. The secondary survey is a head-to-toe examina-tion to identify additional areas of injury.
8. Standard radiographs required for trauma include lateral cervical spine, anteroposterior (AP) chest, and AP pelvis.

OPHTHALMIC TRAUMA

More than one million cases of ophthalmic trauma after penetrating or blunt injury are reported annually in the United States. Prompt and appropriate care of many ophthalmic injuries may prevent much visual disability.

CHEMICAL BURNS

Chemical burns to the eye represent an ophthalmo-logic emergency. If treatment is not begun immediately, irreversible damage may occur. Alkaline substances (i.e., household cleaners, fertilizers, and pesticides) cause the most severe damage, but acids may cause significant ocular morbidity as well.

Treatment

A detailed history is not required before beginning copious irrigation with any available water source for at least 15 to 20 minutes. After initial irrigation, visual acuity and pH should be measured. If the pH has not returned to the normal value of 7.5, irrigation should be continued. Prompt ophthalmologic referral should be obtained in all cases of acid or alkali burns and for patients with decreased visual acuity, severe conjuncti-val swelling, or corneal clouding. All other patients should see an ophthalmologist within 24 hours.

SUPERFICIAL FOREIGN BODIES

Foreign bodies that have an impact on the surface of the cornea or conjunctiva represent approximately 25% of all ocular injuries.

History

An accurate history often provides the diagnosis and should be used to judge the risk of intraocular foreign body (see below). Symptoms range from mild ocular irritation to severe pain. If symptoms began gradually rather than suddenly, other etiologies, such as infectious keratitis, should be considered.

Diagnostic Evaluation

Careful inspection of the cornea and conjunctiva using bright light and magnification often reveals the foreign body.

Treatment

One should always measure visual acuity before making any attempt at removing the foreign body. Superficial foreign bodies can usually be removed using topical anesthesia and a cotton swab. After the foreign body is removed, Wood lamp examination with fluorescein should be performed to ascertain the size of any residual corneal epithelial defect. Eversion of the upper eyelid should be carried out to look for residual foreign material under the lids. Ophthalmologic referral is indicated when a foreign body cannot be safely removed or for any patient with a large corneal epithelial defect.

BLUNT OR PENETRATING INJURY

Blunt or penetrating trauma to the eye represents a leading cause of vision loss in young people. Blunt trauma most often causes ocular contusion or damage to the surrounding orbit. Penetrating trauma causes corneal or scleral laceration (a ruptured globe) and represents an ophthalmologic emergency requiring early intervention and repair. The possibility of a retained intraocular foreign body should always be considered (see below). A high degree of suspicion must be maintained in all cases of head and facial injuries.

History

History should include the mechanism of injury, the force of impact, the likelihood of a retained foreign body, and any associated ocular or visual complaints.

Diagnostic Evaluation

Eyelid integrity, ocular motility, and pupillary reaction should be tested. Use a penlight to detect conjunctival swelling or hemorrhage, corneal or scleral laceration, or hyphema (blood behind the cornea obscuring details of the underlying iris or pupil). Pain and decreased vision with a history of trauma should always lead to suspicion of perforation of the globe. Severe subconjunctival hemorrhage, a shallow anterior chamber or space between the cornea and iris, hyphema, and limitation of extraocular motility are often, but not invariably, present. Radiologic studies, including computed tomography (CT) of the head and orbits, should be obtained in cases of suspected blowout fracture or to rule out a retained intraocular foreign body (see below).

Treatment

If the eye is lacerated or the pupil or iris is not visible, a shield should be placed over the eye, and the patient should be referred immediately to an ophthalmologist. Eyelid lacerations that involve the lid margin or lacrimal apparatus require meticulous repair to avoid severe functional and cosmetic morbidity. If the eyelid margin and inner one sixth of the eyelid are not damaged, the wound can be closed with fine sutures. If the eyelid margin is lacerated, accurate realignment of the lid margin must be ensured before wound closure. Disruption of the inner one sixth of the eyelid requires intubation of the lacrimal drainage system, with stent placement before surgical repair, and should be carried out by an ophthalmologist or other appropriately trained physician. Ophthalmologic referral after trauma is determined by ocular symptoms and findings, as set forth in Table 23-1.

🔑 23-4 KEY POINTS

1. Globe rupture is caused by blunt or penetrating trauma to the eye.
2. A retained foreign body must be ruled out in globe rupture.
3. Simple eyelid lacerations can be repaired once disruption of the lid margin and lacrimal apparatus is excluded.

INTRAOCULAR FOREIGN BODIES

A high-speed missile may penetrate the cornea or sclera while causing minimal symptoms or physical findings. Foreign-body composition is important, because certain metals, such as iron, steel, and copper, produce a severe inflammatory reaction if left in the eye, whereas other materials, such as glass, lead, and stone, are relatively inert and may not require surgical removal. Retained vegetable matter is especially dangerous and may cause a severe purulent endophthalmitis. A retained foreign body should be suspected in all cases of perforating injuries of the eye or whenever the history suggests high-risk activities, such as drilling, sawing, or hammering.

History

One should inquire about high-risk activities, a sensation of sudden impact on the eyelids or eye, and any complaint of pain or decreased vision.

Physical Examination

Visual acuity should always be recorded before any manipulation of the eye or eyelids. Inspection may reveal an entry wound, although this may be quite subtle and easily overlooked. Specifically, one should look for a hyphema, pupillary distortion, or any alteration of the red reflex on funduscopic examination.

Diagnostic Evaluation

Accurate localization may require soft tissue radiographs, orbital ultrasound, or CT. Magnetic resonance imaging is contraindicated in all cases of suspected intraocular foreign body.

Treatment

If the history strongly suggests the possibility of a retained foreign body, urgent ophthalmologic referral is indicated, even in the absence of physical findings.

■ TABLE 23-1 Management of Ophthalmic Trauma
Treat on site and refer immediately
Acid or alkali burn
Unremovable corneal or conjunctival foreign body
Refer immediately
Severe pain
Subnormal visual acuity
Irregular pupil
Deformed globe
Corneal or scleral laceration
Corneal clouding
Severe lid swelling
Severe conjunctival chemosis
Proptosis
Hyphema
Absent red reflex
Suspected intraocular foreign body (history of being struck by high-speed missile)
Eyelid laceration that is deep, large, avulsed, exposes fat, or extends through lid margin or lacrimal drainage apparatus
Refer within 24 hours
Pain
Photophobia
Diplopia
Foreign-body sensation but no visible foreign body or corneal abrasion
Large corneal abrasion
Moderate eyelid or conjunctival chemosis but normal visual acuity
Suspected contusion of globe
Suspected orbital wall fracture
Refer within 48 hours
Mild contusion injury to orbital soft tissues

Prompt surgical removal of intraocular debris is usually indicated to avoid the toxic effect of metallic foreign bodies on intraocular tissue and secondary intraocular infection from retained organic material.

23-5 KEY POINTS

1. Accurate history is the key to correct diagnosis.
2. Magnetic resonance imaging is contraindicated in suspected cases of intraocular foreign body.
3. Surgical removal of foreign bodies is usually indicated.

References

Bell RM, Krantz BE. Initial assessment. In: Moore EE, Feliciano DV, Mattox KL, eds. *Trauma*. New York, NY: McGraw-Hill; 2000:153–170.

Chan O, Walsh M, Wilson A. Major trauma. *BMJ*. 2005;330(7500):1136–1138.

Giuha A. Management of traumatic brain injury. *Postgrad Med J*. 2004;80(949):650–653.

24

Plastic Surgery

Plastic surgery is the repair and reconstruction of bodily deformity due to congenital defects, posttraumatic tissue loss, or postablative defects. By achieving wound closure using local tissue rearrangement or distant tissue transfer, the plastic surgeon strives to restore form and maximize function.

THE RECONSTRUCTIVE LADDER

The various techniques and methods of wound closure can be ordered in a conceptual hierarchy, beginning with the simplest technique to the most complex (Fig. 24-1). The plastic surgeon determines which rung of the ladder is the best initial step for repair of a particular defect based on the complexity of the wound and a thorough evaluation of the patient and his or her clinical situation.

PRIMARY CLOSURE

This is the simplest and most common method of wound closure. Surgical wounds created at the time of an operation are usually closed primarily at the termination of the procedure, typically by using sutures or metal staples. Various suturing techniques can be used, depending on the nature of the wound (see Ch. 1, Fig. 1-6).

After ensuring complete hemostasis within the wound, the skin edges are everted and coapted in a tension-free manner. If tissue injury is minimal and no tissue has been lost, the healing should be rapid and scar formation minimal. If the wound resulted from traumatic injury and is relatively clean without significantly devitalized tissue, primary closure is often performed after thorough wound irrigation with sterile saline solution.

DELAYED PRIMARY CLOSURE

This method of closure is often chosen if the wound is contaminated or requires a period of debridement. Sutures are placed untied between the wound edges at the time of operation, and wound care is performed for several days. The sutures are tied and the wound edges coapted once wound contamination is controlled.

SECONDARY INTENTION

Wounds with heavy bacterial contamination or tissue devitalization requiring debridement are often left open and unsutured. The wound defect gradually fills with beefy red fibrovascular granulation tissue, and epithelialization occurs over time.

GRAFTS

When the degree of tissue loss prevents closure using the above techniques, more sophisticated methods of reconstruction are utilized. Grafting transfers tissue from one site to another. Most grafts are autografts (patient is both donor and recipient), although other types of grafts can be used in certain situations (isograft, allograft, or xenograft). Grafts lack an intrinsic blood supply and must become revascularized at the site of insertion. Material used for grafts includes skin, cartilage, fat, nerve, bone, or tendon.

Skin is the most common tissue graft. Open wounds require barrier reconstitution to prevent bacterial invasion and fluid loss. Skin is harvested as either split-thickness or full-thickness grafts.

Split-thickness skin grafts (STSG) are thin sheets of skin harvested from donor sites; they contain varying amounts of dermis and the overlying epidermis

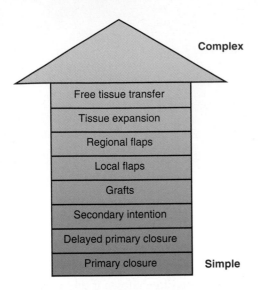

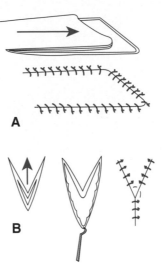

Figure 24-3 • (A) Advancement flap. **(B)** V-Y advancement flap.

Figure 24-1 • The reconstructive ladder.

(Fig. 24-2). The graft is often meshed by creating many tiny incisions, which allow the graft to expand over a larger surface area and better conform to undulating surfaces, while also allowing drainage of underlying wound exudates. The anterior thigh is a common donor site for routine procedures. In patients with extensive burns, however, any undamaged skin is a potential donor site. Donor sites re-epithelialize from epithelial cells remaining within transected hair follicles.

Full-thickness skin grafts (FTSG) contain the entire dermis and epidermis. They are used to close surgical defects when durability, color match, appearance, and lack of wound contraction are required. The groin, flank, and postauricular area are common donor sites. Full-thickness donor sites require primary closure or STSG closure.

LOCAL FLAPS

Local flaps are blocks of tissue that maintain an intrinsic blood supply and are derived from tissue immediately adjacent to the recipient bed. A local tissue flap either advances (V-Y advancement flap, rectangular advancement flap; Fig. 24-3) or pivots (rotation flap or transposition flap; Fig. 24-4).

When dealing with scar contractions that affect a patient's function, plastic surgeons frequently use a Z-plasty technique to gain scar length and to alter the direction of the scar. A Z-plasty is two opposing transposition flaps that switch places and thereby gain length along the central axis of the original Z while also changing its direction by 90 degrees (Fig. 24-5). This extra length diminishes the contracture and improves mobility.

REGIONAL FLAPS

When adjacent tissue is inadequate, a flap is raised from a distant location and inset for defect closure. Flaps include adipocutaneous, fasciocutaneous, myocutaneous, osteocutaneous, or muscular flaps (Fig. 24-6). Once the flap becomes vascularized from the recipient tissue bed, the original vascular pedicle can be transected. The classic operation of this type is the tagliacotian operation—devised by the Italian surgeon Gasparo Tagliacozzi (1546–1599)—in which a forearm flap is transferred to the nose (Italian rhinoplasty). Other examples are groin flaps to the hand and cross

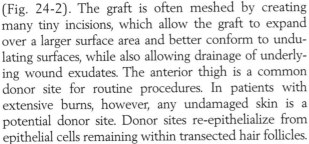

Figure 24-2 • Cross section of skin showing various thickness of split-thickness grafts.

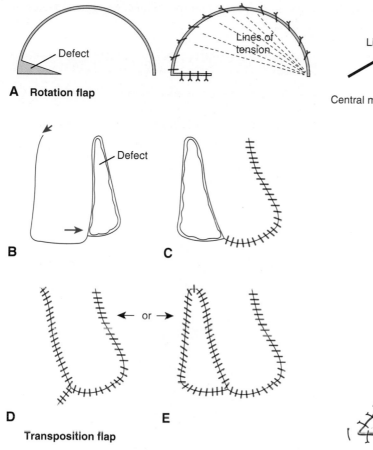

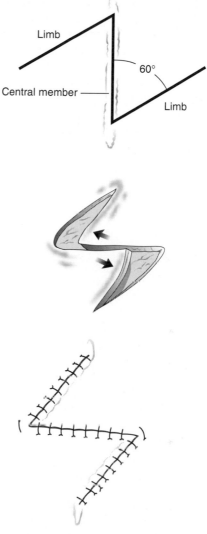

Figure 24-4 • **(A)** Rotation flap. **(B)–(E)** Transposition flap. From Taylor J. *Blueprints Plastic Surgery*. Boston, MA: Blackwell Science; 2004:Fig. 5.

Figure 24-5 • Z-plasty.
Taylor J. *Blueprints Plastic Surgery*. Boston, MA: Blackwell Science; 2004;Fig. 5.

leg flaps. Prolonged awkward positioning is often required postoperatively until the pedicle is eventually transected.

A common pedicled musculocutaneous flap used for breast reconstruction is the transverse rectus abdominis myocutaneous (TRAM) flap. The contralateral rectus abdominis muscle is mobilized, with the superior epigastric artery left intact to supply the large attached skin paddle. The bulky paddle and muscle pedicle are tunneled superiorly and inserted into the breast defect, while the abdominal donor site is closed, resulting in a "tummy tuck" (abdominoplasty; Fig. 24-7).

TISSUE EXPANSION

Silicone balloons are placed under the dermis and gradually inflated over time, causing the overlying soft tissues to "expand." This creates additional surface

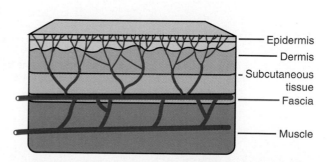

Figure 24-6 • Cross section of soft tissues used for flaps.

area that can be used for breast reconstruction, scalp reconstruction, or any defect requiring local tissue transfer (Fig. 24-8). Benefits of tissue expansion include good skin color match, as well as preservation of hair and sensation.

FREE TISSUE TRANSFER

In free tissue transfer, a tissue block with a feeding nutrient artery is harvested from a distant donor site and transferred to a recipient site, with anastomosis of the nutrient artery to a new blood supply and of the vein to a new venous drainage using microvascular techniques.

🔑 24-1 KEY POINTS

1. Goals of plastic surgery are to restore form and maximize function.
2. Methods of wound closure are based on the principle of the reconstructive ladder.
3. Complex wounds require complex wound closure techniques.

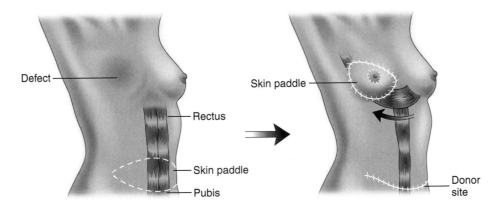

Figure 24-7 • TRAM flap.
TRAM, transverse rectus abdominis myocutaneous.
From Taylor J. *Blueprints Plastic Surgery.* Boston, MA: Blackwell Science; 2004;Fig. 7.

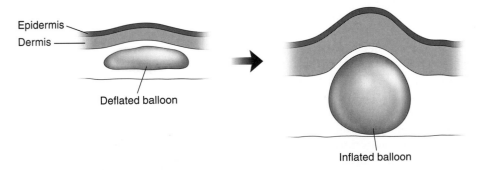

Figure 24-8 • Tissue expansion with silicone balloons.
From Taylor J. *Blueprints Plastic Surgery.* Boston, MA: Blackwell Science; 2004;Fig. 8.

References

Donato, MC. Skin grafting: historic and practical approaches. *Clin Podiatry Med Surg*. 2000; 17(4);561–598.

Goldman GD. Rotation flaps. *Dermatol Surg*. 2005; 31(8 Pt 2):1006–1013.

Levin LS. The reconstructive ladder: an orthoplastic approach. *Orthop Clin North Am*. 1993;24(3):393–409.

OSTEOARTHRITIS

BACKGROUND

Osteoarthritis is the single most common disease of the joints; as such, it is one of the most important causes of morbidity in the United States. Loss of articular cartilage in the synovial joint is the pathologic lesion. This loss can be due to repetitive load-bearing stress or intrinsic properties of either the cartilage or bone or in the body's ability to repair these structures. Joints commonly involved include the interphalangeal, thumb base, hip, knee, and spine. Risk factors include age, obesity, and female sex. Secondary osteoarthritis can occur after major trauma to the joint; repetitive stress; prior inflammatory joint disease; metabolic disease, including ochronosis, hemochromatosis, and Wilson disease; and endocrine disease, including acromegaly, diabetes, and hyperparathyroidism.

HISTORY AND PHYSICAL EXAMINATION

Patients are usually over 55. Typical complaints include a deep ache in the affected joint that is exacerbated by use. Stiffness is common, especially after inactivity, but usually resolves with use. There are no systemic symptoms. Early in the disease, there is little inflammation of the joint, but in later stages, inflammation can be significant.

Physical examination reveals limitation of motion secondary to pain. Localized tenderness and soft tissue swelling may be present. Motion of the joint may produce bony crepitus. As the disease progresses, there may be gross deformities of the joint, with loss of motion.

DIAGNOSTIC EVALUATION

Radiographic examination reveals narrowing of joint spaces. Subchondral bone sclerosis and osteophytes may be present. In primary osteoarthritis, laboratory values are normal. Specific lab tests may be useful to diagnose causes of secondary osteoarthritis. Synovial fluid usually reveals a mononuclear leukocytosis; this test may be useful to exclude other diagnoses, including a septic joint.

TREATMENT

Therapy for osteoarthritis should be based on the severity of the symptoms. In general, exercises to strengthen the joint and preserve or increase range of motion are critical. A cane may dramatically improve mobility. No pharmacologic interventions can reverse the lesions of osteoarthritis, but nonsteroidal anti-inflammatory agents can provide symptomatic relief for pain. Intra-articular steroids can be extremely effective for pain. Hyaluronic acid injection may also be of benefit.

Surgical treatment should be reserved for patients with debilitating pain or compromised quality of life after nonsurgical options are exhausted. In patients with mild disease, osteotomy may produce significant pain relief. Total joint arthroplasty has excellent results in patients with more advanced disease.

JOINT PAIN

It is important to distinguish between acute and chronic causes of pain. Critical questions include history of trauma, swelling, decreased range of motion, and problems with weight bearing. Positions or circumstances that alleviate or exacerbate the pain may yield clues to the diagnosis.

On physical exam, a careful search for swelling, joint effusions, pain on or decreased range of motion, deformity, tenderness, and instability should be made.

KNEE PAIN: COMMON DIAGNOSES

Meniscal Injury

Meniscal injuries are most common in men but can occur in women. Injury to the medial meniscus is more common than to the lateral meniscus. Pain is the most common symptom. Effusions may be present, and weight bearing may be difficult. Exam usually reveals poorly localized tenderness, which may be exacerbated by extension of the joint. A McMurray test may be positive: The knee is placed at 90 degrees and extended while the hip is rotated. A click on medial rotation suggests damage to the lateral meniscus, while discomfort on lateral rotation suggests damage to the medial meniscus.

Magnetic resonance imaging (MRI) is accurate and sensitive for meniscal injury. When confirmed, arthroscopy with meniscectomy is very effective in treating the lesions and has a relatively short recovery time.

Cruciate Ligament Injury

The cruciate ligaments stabilize the knee to translational motion. Acute pain in the setting of trauma and subsequent swelling should alert the examiner to this possibility. Typically, a twist or hyperextension trauma causes these lesions. The pain may improve after the initial injury, but chronic pain may develop. Diagnostic maneuvers include an anterior or posterior drawer sign, in which the knee is flexed 90 degrees, the foot is stabilized on the floor, and pressure is applied to translate the tibia anteriorly or posteriorly. Pain or laxity on anterior motion suggests an anterior ligament injury, while pain or laxity on posterior motion suggests posterior ligament injury.

Treatment is usually conservative, as the ligaments do not heal well and repairs may be unsatisfactory.

Bursitis

Inflammation of the bursa underlying the semimembranosus tendon is a common cause of knee pain in adults. Swelling may be severe, and palpation of the medial aspect of the tibial plateau is usually painful. Conservative treatment is usually effective.

SHOULDER PAIN: COMMON DIAGNOSES

The complexity of the shoulder joint can make diagnosis difficult. A variety of structures can be injured or inflamed, but most problems respond to conservative therapy.

Subacromial Bursitis

This bursa lies lateral and deep to the acromion and can become inflamed with repeated use. Palpation will reveal tenderness. This problem usually responds to conservative therapy with rest and anti-inflammatory agents.

Biceps Tendonitis

The biceps tendon crosses the shoulder joint and may become inflamed where it traverses the bicipital groove. This is best identified on shoulder rotation.

Glenohumeral Pain

The joint itself can become damaged in a variety of ways. Pain may be elicited by palpating over the head of the humerus and rotating the shoulder.

Rotator Cuff Injuries

The rotator cuff is a collection of the tendons of the supraspinatus, infraspinatus, subscapularis, and teres minor. Injury to this structure frequently occurs from trauma or repetitive motion. Forceful abduction of the shoulder against resistance reproduces the pain. It may be difficult to distinguish between inflammation of the cuff and a tear. Inability to elevate the arm after 90 degrees of abduction suggests a tear. MRI is sensitive and specific for rotator cuff injuries. Surgery is an option if conservative measures fail.

BACK PAIN

Back pain is an epidemic in the United States, causing chronic disability in 1% of the population, with a cost of approximately $50 billion annually. Back pain can be divided into local pain that occurs from nerve endings in the vicinity of the lesion; spinal pain, caused by abnormalities of the bony spine; radicular pain, caused by nerve root pathology; and muscle spasm.

The most common causes of back pain include spondylosis, ankylosing spondylitis, disk prolapse, neoplasm, and infection.

Spondylosis

Osteoarthritis of the spine is a common cause of back pain. Symptoms are usually exacerbated by movement and cause limitation of movement, which can be severe. X-rays are helpful, but findings do not necessarily correlate with the radiographic appearance. Lesions include osteophytes, facet hypertrophy, and stenosis of the spinal canal, all of which can cause nerve impingement.

Ankylosing Spondylitis

In contrast to spondylosis, back pain in patients with ankylosing spondylitis is usually worse in the morning and improves with exercise. Patients are usually males who present prior to age 40. Human leukocyte antigen B27 is associated with the disease. Patients will often have an elevated sedimentation rate. The disease is characterized by inflammation and destruction of the bones, which results in ossification of the soft tissues of the spine and fusion of the joints. Fractures may result. Initially, physical therapy and nonsteroidal anti-inflammatory agents are useful. Ultimately, surgery may be required to increase mobility. Typically, surgery is used to repair hip joint arthritis or to correct severe spinal deformity.

Disk Prolapse

A common cause of back pain, this lesion occurs when the nucleus pulposus prolapses through the annulus fibrosis. Posterior prolapse may cause nerve root impingement, whereas anterior prolapse can result in spinal cord impingement. Onset of pain is usually acute and may be associated with tenderness over the nerve root and decreased range of motion in the affected muscles. In the acute setting, it is critical to assess for problems with bowel or bladder function to determine cord compression. MRI is the test of choice to establish the diagnosis. Indications for surgery include muscle weakness, bowel or bladder dysfunction, and incapacitating pain. The benefit of surgery has been questioned when performed for pain alone.

Neoplasm

Metastatic cancer is a common cause of back pain. In this case, the pain tends to be constant and not relieved with either rest or exercise. Plain films usually make the diagnosis, and MRI may be useful to plan palliative treatment.

Infection

Osteomyelitis of the spine most commonly occurs in debilitated patients or intravenous drug abusers and is usually associated with some type of systemic infection. Patients will usually have tenderness at the site and with movement. Pain is typically constant, and signs of systemic infection are present. The sedimentation rate is often elevated. Plain films may be negative initially, MRI is usually diagnostic, and tagged white cell scan may light up the affected area.

HIP FRACTURE

Hip fracture is the most common fracture causing hospital admission. Approximately 300,000 hip fractures occur each year in the United States. The generally advanced age of patients with this problem leads to a staggering 50% 1-year mortality after injury. Three general types of fracture occur: fractures of the femoral neck, intertrochanteric fractures, and subtrochanteric fractures. The first two are by far the most common and usually occur in the elderly as a result of a relatively low-impact type of injury.

Diagnosis is usually made on plain films. In general, because of the possibility of long-term failure of the prosthesis, younger patients should not have primary hip replacement if reduction and fixation are possible. In contrast, hemiarthroplasty may be a good initial choice in the elderly.

🔑 25-1 KEY POINTS

1. Orthopedic injuries are a tremendous cause of economic loss, morbidity, and mortality in the United States.
2. Osteoarthritis is caused by loss of articular cartilage and is best managed conservatively, unless symptoms are debilitating.
3. Causes of knee pain include meniscal injury, cruciate ligament injury, and bursitis. Magnetic resonance imaging is the study of choice to delineate the anatomy and to plan treatment.
4. In the United States, back pain is an epidemic, with an economic cost of $50 billion per year.
5. Conservative therapy for back pain is usually best, unless there are neurologic symptoms or intractable pain.
6. Hip fracture is a common lesion in the elderly and carries high mortality at 1 year.

Reference

Canale ST, ed. *Campbell's Operative Orthopaedics.*
10th ed. St. Louis, MO: Mosby Year-Book (a division
of Elsevier, Inc.); 2002.

Perioperative Care

PREOPERATIVE EVALUATION

Preoperative evaluation has two main purposes: identification of modifiable risk factors and risk assessment. Unless the situation is emergent, every patient should have a detailed history and physical exam. In all patients, attention should be given to a history of cerebrovascular accident, heart disease of any kind, pulmonary disease, renal disease, liver disease and other gastrointestinal disorders, diabetes, prior surgeries, bleeding problems, clotting problems, difficulty with anesthesia, poor nutrition, alcohol use, and illicit drug use. Allergies, current medications, family history, social history, and a careful and complete review of systems should be conducted. Often, the review of systems will reveal problems that require more detailed workup.

Physical examination should be focused on identifying problems that require further workup. For example, cerebrovascular accident may be manifested by facial asymmetry, speech problems, weakness, or a carotid bruit. Cardiac disease may present with evidence of congestive heart failure, crackles on lung exam, or jugular venous distention.

Pulmonary disease may result in, for example, a barrel chest with poor air movement in patients with chronic obstructive pulmonary disease or wheezing in patients with asthma. Liver disease may cause ascites, caput medusae, telangiectasias, or asterixis. Ecchymosis may be evidence of bleeding problems, whereas extremity swelling may result from clotting disorders.

Choice of laboratory studies depends on the patient's underlying medical condition and the extent of the surgery. There has been a trend toward less routine testing and increased reliance on the history and physical exam. In otherwise healthy patients undergoing minor surgery, laboratory studies, including coagulation studies, are probably not indicated. Similarly, in patients with no history of pulmonary or cardiac disease and no significant risk factors undergoing minor or moderate surgery, electrocardiogram (EKG) and chest x-ray (CXR) are also probably not indicated.

General guidelines for preoperative testing in patients without risk factors are as follows:

EKG: Male older than 40 or female older than 50 undergoing cardiovascular procedures

CXR: All patients older than 60 or undergoing thoracic procedures

Hematocrit: All patients if the procedure is expected to cause greater than 500 mL of blood loss

Creatinine: Patients older than 50 or if the procedure has a high risk for generating renal failure

Pregnancy test: All women of childbearing age if pregnancy status is uncertain

Initial preoperative evaluation may suggest additional testing needed, either to determine the surgical risk or to further identify modifiable factors. For example, chest pain or shortness of breath with mild exertion should prompt a more thorough cardiac evaluation, including an EKG and stress test. If these tests show cardiac disease, a decision will need to be made whether the patient requires an intervention prior to the surgery. If preoperative assessment demonstrates carotid artery disease, it may be best to perform an endarterectomy prior to the originally planned surgery. Other issues, such as poorly controlled diabetes, obesity, and malnutrition, should also be addressed prior to surgery. This may involve modifications of diet and insulin dose, weight loss, or inpatient admission for total parenteral nutrition.

Once the risk factors for surgery have been identified, a frank discussion should be held with the patient explaining the potential risks and benefits of the surgery and which risk factors should be addressed prior to the surgery. This discussion should be the basis for the informed consent for surgery. The outcome of this discussion may be that the surgery should proceed without delay or that the procedure is too risky and should not be attempted or somewhere in between. For example, in a young healthy person with a symptomatic inguinal hernia, surgery without delay is indicated. On the other hand, if the hernia is small and asymptomatic and the patient has advanced liver disease with uncontrolled ascites, the risk of the surgery probably outweighs the benefits. In a patient with end-stage renal disease undergoing workup for a kidney transplant who is found to have unstable angina and coronary disease amenable to intervention, the coronary intervention should proceed prior to the transplant.

INTRAOPERATIVE MANAGEMENT

FLUIDS AND ELECTROLYTES

Fluids and electrolytes must be provided in adequate amounts to replace intraoperative losses. This will maintain blood pressure and ensure optimal cardiac function. Choice of fluids depends on the underlying medical problems. For example, the use of potassium-containing fluids should be avoided in patients with renal failure. For longer and more complicated cases, consideration of loss of other electrolytes, including calcium and magnesium, must be addressed.

BLOOD PRODUCTS

Administration of blood products depends on the underlying health of the patient and the type of operation. Whereas in a healthy patient with a limited intraoperative event in which 500 cc of blood are lost, resulting in a hematocrit of 24, a transfusion may not be indicated. However, for a liver transplant patient with expected ongoing blood loss, transfusion may be indicated at a level of 28. Transfusion of fresh frozen plasma and platelets should be considered for patients with coagulopathy or thrombocytopenia.

CARDIAC RISK FACTORS

In patients with known cardiac disease, aggressive intraoperative lowering of myocardial oxygen demand

with beta-blockers has been shown in randomized trials to improve outcomes and should be used.

ANTIBIOTICS

Antibiotics are of benefit in all procedures in which a body cavity is opened and are probably useful in clean procedures. Guidelines for the use of antibiotics include administration prior to the incision (within 1 hour) and redosing after 4 hours. Specific recommendations are shown in Table 26-1.

DIABETES MANAGEMENT

Tight perioperative control of sugars decreases wound infection rates in randomized controlled studies.

TEMPERATURE

Maintenance of normal intraoperative temperature is critical for adequate hemostasis and optimal cardiovascular function. Use of warmed fluids and warming blankets may be necessary for long operations or those in which large body cavities are opened.

POSTOPERATIVE MANAGEMENT

Principles of postoperative management include early mobilization, pulmonary therapy, early nutrition, adequate fluid and electrolyte administration, management of cardiac risk factors, control of blood sugars, and recognition of complications.

■ TABLE 26-1 Antibiotic Recommendations	
Type of Procedure	**Antibiotic Choice**
Clean	Cefazolin or none
Cardiovascular	Cefazolin
Colorectal	Oral: Neomycin/erythromycin base + mechanical cleansing prior to surgery
	Parenteral: cefazolin/Flagyl or cefotetan
Prosthetic Joint	Cefazolin

Early mobilization is important to prevent muscle wasting and weakness, reduce the risk of venous thromboembolism, reduce the rate of pneumonia, and perhaps speed the return of bowel function. If permitted by the type of surgery, the patient should get out of bed on the day of surgery and be walking on the first postoperative day.

One of the most common postoperative complications is pneumonia. Deep-breathing exercises and the use of an incentive spirometer can decrease this risk.

Early nutrition (within 24 hours of surgery) has been demonstrated in randomized controlled trials to improve outcomes. In most patients, this will amount to having them eat, but many patients may require a nasoenteric tube for this purpose. In patients undergoing surgery on gastrointestinal tract, the timing of feeds should be individualized to the patient and the type of operation.

Fluid administration is one of the most important aspects of postoperative care. Adequate resuscitation prevents renal failure and optimizes cardiac function. Excessive fluid can cause congestive heart failure and edema, which in turn inhibits wound healing. Fluid administration must be individualized to the patient and the type of operation: General guidelines are to administer fluid to keep the urine output above 30 cc per hour.

Decreasing cardiac risk requires adequate beta blockade throughout the perioperative period. The heart rate should be kept below 70 and lower if hemodynamically tolerated.

Tight control of blood sugars is clearly beneficial in reducing wound infections. This is accomplished initially by aggressive use of sliding-scale insulin and resumption of the patient's home insulin regimen when the patient is eating adequately.

Early recognition of surgical complications is critical to effectively manage them. Common to all but the most minor operations are wound infections, pneumonia, urinary tract infection, catheter infections, deep venous thrombosis, and myocardial infarction. In addition, each operation has its specific complications. Recognition of a complication depends on detailed daily history and physical exam. Wounds should be examined for erythema and discharge. Particularly worrisome is murky brown discharge that may represent a dehiscence or necrotizing fasciitis. Lungs should be examined daily for decreased breath sounds and egophony, and sputum should be examined. Thick green or brown sputum should prompt investigation for pneumonia, including chest x-ray and sputum gram stain and culture. Sites of catheter placement should be examined for erythema and discharge. Urinary symptoms should prompt a urinalysis and culture. Chest pain in the perioperative period should be taken very seriously and evaluated with an EKG and cardiac enzymes in the appropriate clinical setting.

Evaluation of fever involves the problems discussed above. Other sources of fever include atelectasis, deep venous thrombosis, transfusion reaction, drug reaction, tumor, and pulmonary embolism.

Examples of complications related to the surgery include fascial dehiscence, breakdown or stricture of enteric anastomoses, thrombosis of vascular grafts, deep space infections, and hernia recurrence. These problems can usually be recognized with careful patient examination.

FLUIDS AND ELECTROLYTES

Understanding fluid and electrolyte replacement begins with knowing the composition of the various body compartments. In a typical 70 kg person, 60% of total body weight is water. Two thirds of this water is contained in the intracellular compartment, and one third is in the extracellular compartment. A quarter of this extracellular water is plasma—approximately 3.5 L in a typical man. Red cell volume is about 1.5 L. Combined with plasma, this results in a blood volume of about 5 L. Electrolyte concentrations in the extracellular and intracellular space are as shown in Table 26-2.

Maintenance requirements for healthy adults include urinary fluid loss of 1 L, gastrointestinal loss of 200 mL, and insensible losses of 10 mL/kg. Each of these numbers can be adjusted upward in various disease states. Fever, burns, and diarrhea are examples of processes that can dramatically increase fluid losses.

■ TABLE 26-2 Electrolyte Concentrations in the Extracellular and Intracellular Space		
	Extracellular (mEq/L)	Intracellular (mEq/L)
Sodium	140	10
Potassium	4	150
Calcium	2.5	4.0
Magnesium	1.1	34
Chloride	104	4
Carbonate	24	12
Phosphate	2	40

TABLE 26-3 Normal Replacement of Fluids in Surgical Patients (mEq/L)

Type of Fluid	Sodium	Potassium	H+	Bicarbonate
Gastric	20–120	12	30–100	0
Duodenal	110	15	0	10
Ileum (ileostomy)	100	10	0	40
Colon (diarrhea)	120	25	0	45
Bile	140	5	0	25
Pancreas	140	5	0	115

Normal replacement in surgical patients is 1 mEq/kg of sodium and 0.5 mEq/kg of potassium per day. Gastrointestinal losses in patients can be approximated with the information provided in Table 26-3.

The composition of various replacement fluids is as shown in Table 26-4.

Common electrolyte abnormalities in the perioperative period include hyponatremia, hypernatremia, hyperkalemia, and hypokalemia.

Causes of hyponatremia should be divided into two types, depending on whether there is reduced plasma osmolality. If plasma osmolality is normal or high, the differential diagnosis is hyperlipidemia, hyperproteinemia, hyperglycemia, and mannitol administration. In this case, the treatment focuses on correcting the abnormality in the osmotically active agent.

More common, the plasma osmolality is reduced. In this case, the question becomes whether the circulating plasma volume is high, as in congestive heart failure, cirrhosis, nephrotic syndrome, malnutrition; normal, as in syndrome of inappropriate secretion of ADH, paraneoplastic syndromes, endocrine disorders, and various drugs (morphine, aminophylline, indomethacin); or low, with excessive losses or inadequate replacement.

In general, states with decreased plasma volume should be treated with hypertonic saline if the level is low enough to warrant treatment (<120 mEq/L). In this case, it is critically important to not correct the sodium more than 0.5 mEq/L/hr. If patients are symptomatic, however, it may be advisable to raise the level more quickly. This should only be done in consultation with a neurologist, as faster rates can result in central pontine myelinolysis from the osmotic shift.

States in which the effective plasma volume is high should be treated with fluid restriction.

Causes of hypernatremia are divided into water loss and sodium administration. Water loss can be from insensible losses from infection, burns, or fever; renal loss from diabetes insipidus; gastrointestinal losses; or hypothalamic disorders. Sodium administration can be via ingestion or intravenously. Treatment consists of addressing the underlying abnormality and administering fluid. Correction of hypernatremia should not progress at a rate >0.5 mEq/L/hr, unless neurologic symptoms are present. Rapid correction of hyponatremia can result in seizures, cerebral edema, and death.

Hypokalemia is usually due to potassium loss. Hypokalemia can result in cardiac arrhythmias, especially in patients taking digoxin. Treatment is with exogenous replacement.

Hyperkalemia is usually due to exogenous administration or from intracellular stores. It can result in weakness and cardiac arrhythmias. If the level rises above 6 or the patient has EKG changes, treatment with calcium, insulin, and glucose can transiently decrease plasma potassium, which may rebound, because these treatments do not alter the total body calcium. Kayexalate decreases total body potassium but takes longer to be effective. Dialysis is extremely effective in lowering potassium.

TABLE 26-4 Composition of Various Replacement Fluids (mEq/L)

	Sodium	Potassium	Chloride	Calcium	Lactate
Normal saline	154	154	0	0	0
Half normal saline	77	77	0	0	0
Lactated Ringer	130	4	109	3	28

References

Joehl RJ. Preoperative evaluation: pulmonary, cardiac, renal dysfunction, and comorbidities. *Surg Clin North Am.* 85:6:1061–1073.

Nathens AB, Maier RV. *Surgery: Basic Science and Clinical Evidence.* New York, NY: Springer-Verlag; 2000:151–161.

Appendix: Sample Operative Reports

After each operation, a complete and concise description, outlining the indications for surgery, the operative findings, and the conduct of the operation, should be composed. This report is vital for communication among health care providers, and it documents the intervention for future reference. When dictating a report, follow a defined format, introduce only relevant information to the narrative, and maintain an orderly flow from incision to closure. The following operative reports are examples of routine general surgery procedures: open hernia repair and laparoscopic cholecystectomy.

INGUINAL HERNIA

PREOPERATIVE DIAGNOSIS: Right inguinal hernia
POSTOPERATIVE DIAGNOSIS: Right indirect inguinal hernia
PROCEDURE PERFORMED: Open mesh repair of right indirect inguinal hernia
SURGEON: James Morris, MD
ANESTHESIA: Local and intravenous sedation

INDICATIONS FOR OPERATION: Mr. Robert Hall is a 75-year-old male who presented complaining of a symptomatic right inguinal hernia of 6 months' duration. On physical examination, a nontender reducible right inguinal hernia was noted. Operative and nonoperative management options, as well as the risks and potential complications of each approach, were discussed with the patient. After all questions were answered, he requested open mesh hernia repair. A request-for-surgery form was signed and witnessed preoperatively.

INTRAOPERATIVE FINDINGS: Moderate indirect inguinal hernia sac, ligated and resected. Polypropylene mesh plug inserted into deep ring with mesh overlay.

DESCRIPTION OF PROCEDURE: The patient was positioned supine on the operating table, and preoperative antibiotics and intravenous sedation were administered. The right inguinal region was prepped and draped sterilely. Combined lidocaine 1% and bupivacaine 0.25% was injected subdermally, and an oblique skin incision was made above the inguinal ligament. The superficial epigastric vessels were divided between clamps and tied. The Scarpa fascia was divided and the external oblique fascia identified. A subfascial local anesthetic infiltration was performed, and the external oblique fascia was opened in the line of its fibers down through the external ring. The iliohypogastric nerve was identified and preserved. The ilioinguinal nerve was dissected away from the cord structures

and retracted caudad. Both nerves were preserved and uninjured during the entire procedure. The cord was encircled at the pubic tubercle with a Penrose drain and the floor inspected. There was no evidence of direct herniation; however, the floor was somewhat attenuated. The cord was interrogated, and a moderate-sized indirect hernia sac was identified and dissected free from the surrounding structures. The vas deferens and testicular vessels were preserved and uninjured. Once the proximal sac was fully mobilized into the deep inguinal ring, the distal sac was suture ligated with a 3-0 absorbable stitch and the redundant sac excised and passed off the table as a specimen. A large-sized polypropylene plug was placed into the indirect defect and sutured superiorly for fixation. Given the previously noted attenuated floor, a polypropylene patch was sutured for reinforcement to the conjoined tendon, pubic tubercle, and shelving edge of the inguinal ligament with interrupted 3-0 absorbable suture. The ilioinguinal nerve was returned to its anatomic position alongside the cord structures, and the lateral legs of the patch were positioned around the cord as it exited the deep ring, the legs being secured with a single stitch. The iliohypogastric nerve was then returned to its anatomic position, and the external oblique fascia was closed with a running 3-0 absorbable suture, taking care to avoid entrapment of the ilioinguinal nerve. The Scarpa fascia and then the subdermal layer were reapproximated with interrupted 3-0 absorbable sutures. Skin was further closed with a running 4-0 absorbable subcuticular stitch. Paper reinforcing strips were applied across the incision, followed by a sterile dressing. The patient was then transferred to the recovery room awake and in stable condition. Total intravenous fluids were 300 mL of crystalloid, and blood loss was nil. The only specimen was the hernia sac.

LAPAROSCOPIC CHOLECYSTECTOMY

PREOPERATIVE DIAGNOSIS: Symptomatic cholelithiasis
POSTOPERATIVE DIGAGNOSIS: Same
OPERATION PERFORMED: Laparoscopic cholecystectomy
SURGEON: James Morris, MD
ASSISTANT: Seth Karp, MD
ANESTHESIA: Local, general endotracheal

INDICATIONS FOR OPERATION: Ms. Gloria Brillantes is a 45-year-old female with a 2-year history of episodic postprandial right upper quadrant abdominal pain radiating to the right flank, with associated nausea and occasional emesis. Ultrasonography reveals multiple gallstones with normal gallbladder wall thickness and normal common bile duct caliber. Liver function tests were normal. After surgical consultation and review of her clinical situation, I discussed with the patient the operative and nonoperative management options, including the risks and potential complications of each approach. After all questions were answered, she requested laparoscopic cholecystectomy. A request-for-surgery form was signed and witnessed preoperatively.

INTRAOPERATIVE FINDINGS: Normal-appearing, thin-walled gallbladder without adhesions containing multiple small 5 mm cholesterol gallstones. Liver, stomach, and small and large intestines were grossly normal.

DESCRIPTION OF PROCEDURE: The patient was positioned supine on the operating room table, and preoperative antibiotics and general endotracheal anesthesia were administered. The abdomen was prepped and draped sterilely. The Veress needle was inserted uneventfully through a tiny subumbilical incision, after skin infiltration with combined lidocaine 1% and bupivacaine 0.25%. The abdomen was insufflated with carbon dioxide to 15 mm Hg pressure. A 5 mm port was then placed subumbilically and the 5 mm 30-degree endoscope inserted. The abdomen was inspected and appeared grossly normal. Under additional local anesthesia, a 10 mm port was placed in the epigastric region, and two more 5 mm ports were placed further laterally on the right. The table was placed in reverse Trendelenburg position, with mild rotation to the patient's left side. The gallbladder fundus was retracted cephalad, and the infundibulum was retracted toward the right lower quadrant. Using careful blunt dissection, normal biliary anatomy was encountered. The cystic duct and the artery were easily identified and divided between surgical clips. The gallbladder was then dissected out of the fossa using electrocautery, removed from the abdomen via the epigastric port, and passed off the table as a specimen. The operative field was then inspected and found to be hemostatic and without bile leak. Intact clips were again seen securing the duct and artery stumps. All trocars were then removed under vision, and no port site bleeding was noted. The 10 mm epigastric fascial defect was closed with a figure-of-eight 0 absorbable suture, and all skin incisions were closed with buried simple 4-0 absorbable sutures. Paper reinforcing strips were applied to the incisions, followed by sterile dressings. The patient was uneventfully extubated and transferred to the recovery room in stable condition. Administered intravenous fluids were 500 mL of crystalloid, and blood loss was negligible. Specimens included the gallbladder and contained stones.

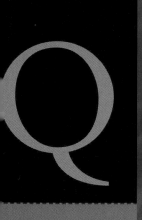

Questions

1. A 71-year-old man with sudden onset of severe abdominal and back pain is brought to the emergency department for evaluation. He has a history of hypertension. He weighs 300 lb. He has a 45-pack-a-year history of smoking. Physical examination reveals a pulsatile abdominal mass. Both lower extremities reveal pallor with diminished pedal pulses. What is the most likely etiology of this patient's condition?
   a. Atherosclerosis
   b. Marfan syndrome
   c. Meningococcal infection
   d. Syphilis
   e. Trauma

2. A 78-year-old man is brought to the emergency department with a 12-hour history of abdominal pain, diarrhea, and vomiting. He has a history of atrial fibrillation and was previously treated for congestive heart failure with digoxin. Physical examination reveals a distended abdomen with significant guarding. Rectal examination reveals guaiac positive stool in the vault. White blood cell count is 24,000/mm³. Abdominal x-ray reveals edema of the bowel wall. What is the most appropriate treatment for this patient?
   a. Angiographic embolization
   b. Antibiotic therapy with ampicillin and gentamicin
   c. Antibiotic therapy with gentamicin
   d. Heparinization followed by oral warfarin
   e. Surgical exploration

3. A 20-year-old male tennis player crashes into a fence trying to chase a ball he thought he could catch up to during an important match. His right knee sustains the brunt of injury. Physical examination reveals edema and decreased range of motion of the knee in flexion and extension. Magnetic resonance imaging (MRI) is performed and reveals dislocation of the joint. No pulse is palpable behind the knee joint. What is the most likely explanation for this finding?

   a. Anterior tibial artery rupture
   b. Peroneal artery hematoma
   c. Popliteal artery spasm
   d. Posterior tibial artery hematoma
   e. Superficial femoral artery spasm

4. A 25-year-old woman found a lump in her right breast on self-examination. She has no family history of breast cancer. The lump is freely mobile and well circumscribed. What is the best option to evaluate a breast mass in a young female?
   a. Biopsy
   b. Mammography
   c. Testing for breast cancer (BRCA) gene
   d. Ultrasound
   e. Watchful waiting

5. A 19-year-old woman began breast-feeding for the first time. At first, it was difficult for her infant to feed. Now, her breasts are red, warm, and sore. She has continued to breast-feed, despite the pain; however, she has recently begun to use a breast pump instead of breast-feeding. She is begun on a course of oral antibiotics. What condition is this patient at risk of developing?
   a. Breast abscess
   b. Fibrocystic disease
   c. Inflammatory breast cancer
   d. Prolactinoma
   e. Tuberculosis

6. A 31-year-old premenopausal woman with a left breast mass undergoes a left modified radical mastectomy. Pathology reveals infiltrating ductal carcinoma measuring 3 cm in size with negative lymph nodes. Estrogen receptor status is negative. What is the most appropriate adjuvant therapy for this patient?
   a. Chemotherapy (multiagent)
   b. External beam radiotherapy

c. High-energy focused ultrasound therapy

d. Tamoxifen

e. Watchful waiting

7. A 31-year-old woman complains of a 6-month history of bloody diarrhea, abdominal pain, and intermittent fevers. She has a history of irritable bowel syndrome but has had a worsening of her symptoms during the above time period. Her past medical history is unremarkable. Physical examination reveals abdominal distension. Bowel sounds are present in all quadrants. Rectal examination reveals multiple anal fissures. What is the most appropriate diagnostic testing for this patient?

a. Anoscopy

b. Colonoscopy

c. Flexible sigmoidoscopy

d. Rigid sigmoidoscopy

e. No further diagnostic testing is required for this patient.

8. A 71-year-old woman presents to her primary care physician complaining of rectal bleeding. She had some mild left-sided abdominal cramps that subsided within a few minutes. She has never had a prior episode of rectal bleeding. Physical examination reveals mild left lower quadrant abdominal pain without evidence of guarding or rebound tenderness. Rectal examination reveals no fresh blood in the rectal vault. Colonoscopy reveals several outpouchings of the sigmoid colon wall without evidence of bleeding or perforation. The remainder of the colonoscopy is within normal limits. White blood cell count is normal. What is the most appropriate treatment for this patient?

a. Antibiotic therapy with ampicillin and gentamicin

b. Left hemicolectomy

c. Right hemicolectomy

d. Subtotal colectomy

e. Watchful waiting

9. An 85-year-old man is brought to the emergency department because of acute abdominal pain and progressive abdominal distention. He is a resident of a local nursing home. He has not been eating because of progressive nausea. Abdominal radiographs reveal a massively sigmoid colon. What is the initial treatment for this patient?

a. Gastrografin enema

b. High-fiber diet

c. Lactulose

d. Rectal tube decompression

e. Surgical resection

10. A 41-year-old woman complains of constant headaches for the past 6 months. She has also complained of female infertility and has been unable to have children, despite having unprotected sexual intercourse with her husband during the past 15 years. Physical examination reveals

deficits in the extraocular movements bilaterally. Breast examination reveals bilateral female gynecomastia. Which of the following laboratory tests would be most useful in diagnosing this patient?

a. Ferritin

b. Hemoglobin

c. Hematocrit

d. Iron

e. Prolactin

11. A 41-year-old woman with Crohn disease has undergone multiple surgical procedures. She has recently undergone an ileostomy but still has evidence of some distal jejunal disease. Her current medications include prednisone and aminosalicylic acid. Which of the following effects of prolonged therapy with glucocorticoids are possible for this patient?

a. Antibody production

b. Collagen formation

c. Fibroblast dysfunction

d. Inflammatory cell migration

e. Wound healing

12. A 49-year-old obese man presents to his primary care physician for a follow-up examination. He has a history of uncontrolled diabetes mellitus and bipolar disorder. His current medications include lithium and milk of magnesium. Physical examination of the heart, lungs, and abdomen are within normal limits. Laboratory studies reveal serum calcium of 14 mg/dL. What is the most likely explanation for these findings?

a. Dietary indiscretion

b. Medication overdose

c. Milk-alkali syndrome

d. Parathyroid adenoma

e. Parathyroid hyperplasia

13. A 41-year-old man has chronic gastroesophageal reflux. He is currently managed with an H_2-blocker. Physical examination of the heart, lungs, and abdomen are within normal limits. Which of the following factors would be least protective of the esophagus in terms of the continued exposure induced by this condition?

a. Arcuate ligament

b. Gastric emptying ability

c. Gravitational effect

d. Salivary gland secretory products

e. Secondary peristaltic waves

14. A 40-year-old woman complains of chest pain and dysphagia to solids. She presents to a specialist for evaluation. Esophageal manometric studies are performed and reveal high-amplitude contractions and eventual normal relaxation of the lower esophageal sphincter. Barium swallow is

normal. What is the most likely diagnosis?

a. Cricopharyngeal muscle spasm
b. Diffuse esophageal spasm
c. Scleroderma
d. Tuberculosis
e. Psychogenic swallowing disorder

15. A 5-year-old boy is brought to the emergency department after ingesting liquid drain cleaner. The boy was left unattended while his baby-sitter was on the telephone. The boy is hoarse and has obvious stridor. What is the most appropriate initial treatment for this patient?

a. Antibiotics
b. Corticosteroids
c. Induction of vomiting with ipecac
d. Placement of nasogastric tube and lavage
e. Tracheostomy

16. A 76-year-old man with a history of vague right upper quadrant pain, a 25 lb weight loss, and anorexia presents to his primary care physician for evaluation. Physical examination reveals scleral icterus. Abdominal examination reveals a right upper quadrant mass. Kidney, ureter, and bladder (KUB) reveals a circular calcification in the right upper quadrant. Exploratory laparotomy reveals a neoplastic process involving the gallbladder and liver. What is the most likely pathology causing this condition?

a. Adenocarcinoma
b. Sarcoma
c. Squamous cell carcinoma
d. Transitional cell carcinoma
e. Tuberculosis granuloma

17. A 38-year-old woman presents to her primary care physician for evaluation of intermittent vague right upper quadrant pain. She has a history of hypothyroidism and hypertension. Her current medications include synthetic thyroid hormone replacement and a calcium channel blocker. Physical examination reveals mild right upper quadrant pain to deep palpation. Ultrasound reveals a 3 cm gallstone. What is the most likely type of stone to be present in this patient?

a. Black gallstone
b. Brown gallstone
c. Calcium oxalate gallstone
d. Type I cholesterol stone
e. Type II cholesterol stone

18. A 46-year-old woman presents to the emergency department complaining of right upper quadrant and a fever to 102°F. Physical examination reveals scleral icterus and significant right upper quadrant pain to palpation. Peritoneal signs are absent. Bowel sounds are present. Which of the following should be included in the initial treatment of this patient?

a. Antibiotics
b. Choledochojejunostomy
c. Decompression with T-tube
d. Endoscopic sphincterotomy
e. Percutaneous transhepatic drainage

19. A 17-year-old boy is brought to the emergency department after suffering from chest pain and dyspnea during a pickup basketball game. Physical examination reveals a systolic crescendo-decrescendo murmur, heard best at the second right intercostal space. The murmur radiates to the right carotid artery. Chest x-ray reveals a normal heart size. Which of the following findings would be expected to be seen on an electrocardiogram in this patient?

a. Inversion of T waves in leads V1–V4
b. Left ventricular hypertrophy
c. Right bundle branch block
d. Right ventricular hypertrophy
e. Right atrial hypertrophy

20. A 72-year-old man collapses while walking in a shopping mall. He is pulseless and apneic. There is no history of trauma. Cardiopulmonary resuscitation (CPR) is started until rescue squad arrives. Advanced cardiac life support (ACLS) protocol is initiated. He is pronounced dead 40 minutes later. Autopsy reveals myocardial necrosis with rupture of the left ventricle. Which of the following is the most likely risk factor that contributed to his death?

a. Family history of diabetes mellitus
b. Hypotension
c. Obesity
d. Sedentary lifestyle
e. Trauma

21. A 57-year-old man is brought to the emergency department complaining of dyspnea and chest pain. He also admits to a 20 lb weight loss. He complains of fevers, chills, and night sweats. Physical examination reveals supraclavicular adenopathy. Chest examination reveals distant heart sounds. Laboratory studies reveal a white blood cell count of 170,000/mm^3. Chest x-ray and echocardiography reveal a pericardial effusion. What is the most likely explanation of these findings?

a. Atrial myxoma
b. Atrial fibrillation
c. Lymphoma
d. Metastatic colorectal carcinoma
e. Pericarditis

22. A newborn male has an opening of the abdominal wall at the umbilicus. He has no other prior medical or surgical history. Birth history was unremarkable. During the remainder of the physical examination and diagnostic testing, which of the following findings may be possible in this patient?

a. Cleft lip
b. Cleft palate
c. Diaphragmatic hernia
d. Pericardium
e. Urinary bladder in retroperitoneum

23. A 44-year-old male construction worker undergoes a right inguinal hernia repair. The surgical procedure is uneventful. He has no prior medical or surgical history. He returns for follow-up on postoperative day 3 for a wound check. The wound is clean, dry, and intact. What is the optimal convalescent period required before returning to work for this patient?
    a. 1 week
    b. 4 weeks
    c. 6 to 8 weeks
    d. 12 weeks
    e. Unknown

24. A 40-year-old woman undergoes repair of a right femoral hernia. During the procedure, the femoral canal is dissected. The anatomic boundaries of the femoral canal include which of the following?
    a. Cooper ligament
    b. Inguinal ligament
    c. Ischial spine
    d. Lacunar ligament
    e. Nerve (femoral)

25. A 53-year-old man undergoes a radical prostatectomy for presumed organ-confined prostate cancer. The most important factor in maintaining continence after radical prostatectomy is preservation of the:
    a. Bladder neck
    b. External urethral sphincter
    c. Levator ani muscle complex
    d. Nervi erigentes
    e. Puboprostatic ligaments

26. A 27-year-old man has bulky retroperitoneal adenopathy following radical orchiectomy for a mixed germ cell tumor. His chest x-ray is normal. Serum beta-human chorionic gonadotropin (β-hCG) and alpha-fetoprotein (AFP) are markedly elevated. Liver enzymes are slightly elevated, and the patient relates a history of ethanol excess. He receives three cycles of chemotherapy. Restaging reveals a 3 cm retroperitoneal mass, a normal chest x-ray, and normal serum β-hCG. However, the serum AFP is 20 IU/ml (normal = 0–9). What is the next step in the management of this patient?
    a. Computed tomography (CT)-guided needle biopsy
    b. External beam radiotherapy
    c. Retroperitoneal lymph node dissection
    d. Salvage chemotherapy
    e. Serial markers and CT scans

27. A 63-year-old man is disease-free two years after bacillus Calmette-Guerin (BCG) therapy for carcinoma in situ (CIS) and a grade 2, stage T1 bladder cancer. In addition to physical examination, cystoscopy, and urinary cytology, evaluation at this time should include:
    a. Intravenous pyelogram
    b. Prostatic urethral biopsy
    c. Random biopsies of the bladder
    d. Selective upper tract cytology
    e. Urinary voided cytology, repeated 3 times

28. A 78-year-old man presents to the emergency department for evaluation of progressive right upper quadrant pain, nausea, vomiting, and a 30 lb weight loss in the past 3 months. He has a prior medical history of cholelithiasis, diabetes mellitus, hypertension, and dementia. Physical examination reveals scleral icterus bilaterally. Abdominal examination reveals right upper quadrant tenderness and a palpable mass. Peritoneal signs are absent. CT scan reveals pancreatic, duodenal, and choledochal lymph nodes. There is an asymmetric thickening of the gallbladder. What is the most likely pathologic finding at exploratory laparotomy and biopsy?
    a. Adenocarcinoma
    b. Fibroma
    c. Lipoma
    d. Myxoma
    e. Myoma

29. An 8-year-old boy undergoes a right upper quadrant ultrasound for persistent right upper quadrant discomfort. He has no prior medical or surgical history. He has no known allergies and takes no medications. His mother has a history of gallstones. Ultrasound findings include a fusiform dilation of the common bile duct. What is the most likely explanation for these findings?
    a. Type I choledochal cyst
    b. Type II choledochal cyst
    c. Type III choledochal cyst
    d. Type IV choledochal cyst
    e. Type V choledochal cyst

30. An 18-year-old man is stabbed in his abdomen multiple times by an assailant during an altercation involving sale of illicit drugs. He is brought to the emergency department for evaluation. He has four stab wounds of the abdomen—three are in the right upper quadrant, and one is in the left lower quadrant. Physical examination of the abdomen reveals guarding and rebound tenderness. The patient is brought to surgery for an exploratory laparotomy. A penetrating injury to the gallbladder is found. Which of the following associated viscera are likely to be injured?
    a. Aorta
    b. Colon

c. Kidney

d. Liver

e. Urinary bladder

31. A 62-year-old woman presents to her primary care physician with a cough. She also complains of hemoptysis. Social history reveals a 55-pack-a-year history of smoking. She is a recovering alcoholic. Physical examination reveals bilateral wheezes. Cardiac, pulmonary, and abdominal examinations are unremarkable. Laboratory values reveal serum calcium of 13 mg/dL. Serum protein electrophoresis shows no abnormal spikes. What is the most likely diagnosis?

a. Goodpasture syndrome

b. Myeloma

c. Renal adenoma

d. Small cell carcinoma of the lung

e. Squamous cell carcinoma of the lung

32. A 10-year-old boy is brought to his primary care physician for evaluation of persistent hoarseness. He has just begun to participate with his school chorus and notes that his hoarseness worsens with singing. Physical examination of the heart, lungs, and abdomen are unremarkable. Fiber optic flexible laryngeal examination reveals multiple lesions on his true vocal cords. What is the most likely diagnosis?

a. Gastroesophageal reflux

b. Granulomatous inflammation of the pharynx

c. Laryngeal papilloma

d. Singer's nodule

e. Thyroid carcinoma

33. A 75-year-old man presents to his primary care physician because of hoarseness. He has a 60-pack-a-year history of smoking. He also complains of a 25 lb weight loss over the past 4 months. Direct laryngoscopy reveals a sessile mass on the high right vocal cord. He also has a palpable lymph node along the right anterior cervical lymph node chain. If dysplasia is found on biopsy of the laryngeal lesion, what is the most likely diagnosis?

a. Adenoma

b. Laryngeal polyp

c. Laryngitis

d. Mucoepidermoid cystic disease

e. Squamous cell carcinoma

34. A 21-year-old male college student presents to the outpatient clinic for a routine examination at the beginning of the fall semester. He has a history of irritable bowel syndrome. Physical examination of the heart, lungs, and abdomen are unremarkable. Genitourinary examination reveals that the testes are descended bilaterally. A left grade I varicocele is present. There are no testicular masses. The penis is uncircumcised, and the foreskin is unable to be retracted behind the glans. What is the most likely diagnosis?

a. Balanitis

b. Hypospadias

c. Epispadias

d. Paraphimosis

e. Phimosis

35. A 71-year-old white male presents to his primary care physician complaining of a 1-month history of nocturia, polyuria and difficulty starting and stopping his urinary stream. His American Urological Association Symptom Score (AUA-IPSS) is 17/35. Physical examination of the prostate reveals an enlarged gland without masses. His testes are descended bilaterally. He has a small right hydrocele that transilluminates. His prostate-specific antigen (PSA) is 6 ng/mL, and urinalysis is negative. The patient is begun on dutasteride 0.5 mg daily. What is a likely result of taking this medication?

a. Ejaculatory dysfunction

b. Maximal change in urinary flow rate

c. Prostate size decreases by 25%

d. Serum PSA increases by 50%

e. Symptom score remains unchanged

36. A 34-year-old white male has a painless enlargement of his right testis in the past 4 months. He is brought to his primary care physician by his girlfriend, who urges him to seek evaluation. He has recently become depressed because of this problem. He had a cryptorchid right testis as an infant, which was surgically corrected. A scrotal ultrasound confirms the presence of a 3 cm hypoechoic right testicular mass. What is the most likely diagnosis?

a. Choriocarcinoma

b. Embryonal (mixed germ cell) carcinoma

c. Endodermal (yolk sac) tumor

d. Seminoma

e. Teratoma

37. A 51-year-old man is found to have an intracranial mass and will undergo resection. The surgical procedure is performed via a transoccipital approach. In this approach, the patient develops a cerebrospinal fluid (CSF) leak. Which of the following statements is true regarding CSF?

a. Arachnoid villi act as two-way valves.

b. Arachnoid villi open at a pressure of 5 mm Hg.

c. CSF is absorbed through the spinal roots.

d. CSF enters through the foramen of Magendie.

e. Total CSF volume is 150 L.

38. A 19-year-old college student is driving under the influence of alcohol, despite recommendations from friends not to drive. She is struck by another driver. The force of impact causes her to strike the temporal area of her skull against the window. She develops a mild headache but does not lose consciousness. Several hours later, she develops a severe headache with nausea and vomiting. Which is the most likely diagnosis?

a. Bacterial infection
b. Berry aneurysm
c. Epidural hematoma
d. Subarachnoid hematoma
e. Subdural hemorrhage

39. A 59-year-old man presents to his primary care physician complaining of progressive right-sided hearing loss and gait unsteadiness. He states that when he uses the phone, he must use his left ear to listen instead of his right ear. He has a past medical history of hypertension. His current medications include a calcium channel blocker. Physical examination reveals loss of the right corneal reflex and facial weakness. Cardiac, pulmonary, and abdominal examinations are within normal limits. What is the most appropriate next best step in the diagnosis of this patient?
a. Audiometric testing
b. Brainstem-evoked potential testing
c. CT scan of the head without contrast
d. MRI of the head
e. Nystagmography

40. A 47-year-old man with a history of end-stage pulmonary disease of his right lung is scheduled for a lung transplant. Preoperative cardiac function is good. He has no history of congenital defects. Which of the following is the most appropriate surgical incision for this patient to have?
a. Chevron abdominal
b. Lateral thoracotomy
c. Midline abdominal
d. Transverse anterior thoracotomy
e. Pfannenstiel

41. A 47-year-old man with multiple medical problems and end-stage pulmonary parenchymal disease undergoes a lung transplant. He has a prior medical history of obstructive lung disease. He has an uncle with cystic fibrosis. His father has restrictive lung disease, and his brother has pulmonary hypertension. Which of the following portends the best survival following lung transplant for this patient?
a. Bronchogenic carcinoma
b. Cystic fibrosis
c. Obstructive lung disease
d. Pulmonary hypertension
e. Restrictive lung disease

42. A 4-year-old boy is on the waiting list for a liver transplant. He has end-stage hepatic disease and is currently hospitalized for esophageal variceal hemorrhage. What is the most likely cause of liver failure in this patient?
a. Biliary atresia
b. Hepatitis A

c. Primary biliary cirrhosis
d. Primary sclerosing cholangitis
e. Tuberculosis

43. A 23-year-old woman who complains of greasy and odorous stools, generalized weakness, and hair loss presents to her primary care physician for evaluation. Physical examination of the heart, lungs, and abdomen are unremarkable. She has no guarding or rebound tenderness. Bowel sounds are present in all quadrants. Female pelvic examination was deferred at the patient's request. What is the most likely explanation of these findings?
a. Gastric ulcer with bleeding
b. Glucose malabsorption
c. Menstruation
d. Pancreatic insufficiency
e. Pituitary tumor

44. A 27-year-old woman is 12 hours status post cadaveric pancreas transplant and currently in the surgical intensive care unit. She has a medical history of insulin-dependent diabetes since age 5. Her vital signs are normal. Chest is clear to auscultation, and cardiac examination reveals a regular rate with a regular rhythm. Wound dressing is clean, dry, and intact. Which of the following is the best method of monitoring the transplanted pancreas?
a. Serum amylase level
b. Serum glucose level
c. Serum insulin level
d. Ultrasonography of the pancreatic vessels
e. Urinary amylase level

45. A 44-year-old man with recurrent pancreatitis is brought to the emergency department with another bout of pancreatitis. Which of the following is the most reassuring factors regarding the severity of his condition?
a. Age
b. Blood glucose level of 300 mg/dL
c. Lactate dehydrogenase level of 400 IU/L
d. Serum calcium of 6 mg/dL
e. Serum hematocrit level of 29%

46. A 41-year-old man with a long history of renal stones and hypercalcemia is found to have an adenoma of the right superior parathyroid gland. He is going to undergo surgical excision of this lesion. What is the best surgical landmark for this lesion?
a. Bifurcation of the carotid arteries
b. Carotid sinus
c. Junction of the inferior thyroid artery and recurrent laryngeal nerve
d. Junction of the upper and middle third of the thyroid gland
e. Recurrent laryngeal nerve

47. Which of the following techniques is best utilized to define an enlarged parathyroid gland?
    a. CT scan of the neck
    b. Dual tracer imaging
    c. MRI of the neck
    d. Thyrocervical angiography
    e. Ultrasonography

48. A 44-year-old man with end-stage renal disease successfully undergoes a renal transplant. He has a prior medical history of hyperparathyroidism. Six months after renal transplantation, his serum calcium is still 13 mg/dL. Which of the following laboratory findings are possible in this patient?
    a. Elevated serum phosphate
    b. Elevated serum lactic acid dehydrogenase
    c. Elevated urine calcium
    d. Elevated urine creatinine
    e. Elevated urine protein

49. A 46-year-old man presents to his primary care physician for evaluation of a skin lesion. He complains of hypopigmentation of the skin of his lower back. He has a prior medical history of eczema and basal cell carcinoma. He is a farmer who spends a great deal of time outdoors. What cells are responsible for this condition?
    a. Adipocytes
    b. Keratin-producing cells
    c. Langerhans cells
    d. Melanocytes
    e. Merkel cells

50. A 69-year-old male presents to his dermatologist with a lesion present on his nose. He is a gardener who spends a great deal of his time outdoors. He has a prior medical history of allergic rhinitis, hypertension, and diabetes mellitus. His current medications include a beta-blocker and an oral hypoglycemic. Physical examination of his nose reveals a raised, shiny, papular lesion with small blood vessels. What is the most likely diagnosis?
    a. Basal cell carcinoma
    b. Histiocytosis X
    c. Melanoma
    d. Seborrheic keratosis
    e. Squamous cell carcinoma

51. A 29-year-old Black woman presents to her primary care physician because of a growth on her left ear, which occurred after she had her ear pierced for the first time a week ago. She noticed that her ear seemed to develop a growth on it quite rapidly. She had never had her ear pierced before. What is the most likely explanation for these findings?
    a. Basal cell carcinoma
    b. Blue nevus

c. Juvenile melanoma
d. Keloid
e. Molluscum contagiosum

52. A 52-year-old Asian American female has melanotic pigmentation of the buccal mucosa, lips, and digits. Colonoscopy reveals hamartomas throughout the gastrointestinal tract. The polyps were removed due to her increased risk of cancer. What other cancer is associated with this condition?
    a. Cervical cancer
    b. Kidney cancer
    c. Liver cancer
    d. Ovarian cancer
    e. Pancreatic cancer

53. A 45-year-old female complains of chronic diarrhea and sweating. Colonoscopy is performed, and a biopsy of a lesion in her ileum is performed. The pathology report shows that the tumor is composed of neuroendocrine cells. What is a medical treatment for this condition?
    a. Corticosteroids, intravenous
    b. Corticosteroids, topical
    c. Furosemide
    d. Octreotide
    e. Tetracycline

54. An 18-year-old male is brought to the emergency department with sudden excruciating abdominal pain localized to the right lower quadrant, nausea and vomiting, mild fever, and slight tachycardia. He has a prior medical history of recurrent otitis media. Physical exam reveals marked right lower rebound tenderness and guarding. Serum white blood cell count is 18,000/mm^3. KUB x-ray reveals bowel gas in the small and large bowel. What is the most likely diagnosis?
    a. Appendicitis
    b. Crohn disease
    c. Diverticulitis
    d. Pancreatitis
    e. Ulcerative colitis

55. A 39-year-old woman presents to the emergency department complaining of severe abdominal pain. She has a history of peptic ulcer disease. Physical examination reveals guarding and rebound tenderness. She is taken to the operating room for exploratory laparotomy. During the procedure, the surgeon who opens the gastrosplenic ligament to reach the lesser sac accidentally cuts an artery. Which of the following vessels is the most likely one injured?
    a. Gastroduodenal artery
    b. Left gastric artery
    c. Left gastroepiploic artery
    d. Right gastric artery
    e. Splenic artery

56. A 2-year-old female is brought to the emergency department because of several episodes of rectal bleeding. A technetium-99 m perfusion scan reveals a 3 cm ileal outpouching located 50 cm from the ileocecal valve. Which of the following types of ectopic tissue does this structure most likely contain?
a. Duodenal
b. Esophageal
c. Gastric
d. Hepatic
e. Jejunal

57. A 39-year-old woman complains of epigastric pain with eating over the past 3 or 4 months. She admits to a history of chronic back problems. She notes weight gain of 20 lb in the past 4 months. She denies the use of nonsteroidal anti-inflammatory agents. She denies nausea and vomiting. Physical examination of the heart, lungs, and abdomen are within normal limits. What is the most likely pathogen associated with this condition?
a. Enterohemorrhagic *Escherichia coli*
b. *Escherichia coli*
c. *Helicobacter pylori*
d. *Shigella sonnei*
e. *Streptococcus pyogenes*

58. A 59-year-old man was injured in a car accident. An abdominal CT scan reveals a ruptured spleen. His blood pressure is 90/40 mm Hg, and his pulse is 140 beats per minute. The patient is taken for laparotomy. Splenectomy is performed. Which of the following laboratory abnormalities is likely after this procedure?
a. Anemia
b Basophilia
c. Eosinophilia
d. Thrombocytopenia
e. Thrombocytosis

59. A 19-year-old man was kicked in the abdomen during a fight in a bar. He went to his primary care physician, who ordered a CT scan, which revealed a subcapsular splenic hematoma. The man was told to restrict physical activity. Two weeks later, he presents to the emergency department because of severe abdominal pain. He undergoes a splenectomy. Postoperatively, a peripheral smear is ordered. Which type of cell can be found in this patient?
a. Basophilic stippling
b. Blister cells
c. Howell-Jolly bodies
d. Nucleated red blood cells
e. Spherocytes

60. A 15-year-old African American male underwent a splenectomy after sustaining a knife injury during a fight. He presents to his primary care physician for a sports physical.

His mother read on the Web that he is at increased risk for infection. He should receive which of the following vaccines to prevent serious infections?
a. *Haemophilus influenzae*
b. Pneumococcus
c. Tetanus
d. Vaccines against common encapsulated organisms
e. Varicella

61. A 53-year-old woman presents to her primary care physician with a 12-month history of neck pain. She complains of a 15-lb weight gain and generalized malaise. She has a past medical history of hypertension and diabetes mellitus. Her current medications include an oral hypoglycemic. Physical examination reveals tenderness along the course of the thyroid gland without evidence of a discrete mass. What is the most likely diagnosis?
a. Acute thyroiditis
b. Hashimoto thyroiditis
c. Papillary thyroid carcinoma
d. Riedel thyroiditis
e. Subacute thyroiditis

62. A 47-year-old woman with a history of a left thyroid mass undergoes left thyroid lobectomy. Pathology reveals a 1.3 cm papillary carcinoma with no evidence of extracapsular extension. What is the most appropriate next step in the treatment of this patient?
a. External beam radiotherapy
b. Multiagent chemotherapy
c. Subtotal thyroidectomy
d. Total thyroidectomy
e. Watchful waiting with periodic follow-up

63. A 34-year-old man with a thyroid nodule is undergoing a neck exploration. During the procedure, it is possible that he will undergo thyroidectomy. Which of the following statements about the superior laryngeal nerve and the innervation of the thyroid gland is correct?
a. Injury to the nerve causes bowing of the vocal cords during phonation.
b. Nerve injury may be unnoticeable in singers.
c. The nerve is rarely at risk during thyroid surgical procedures.
d. The superior laryngeal nerve is chiefly a motor nerve.
e. The superior laryngeal nerve is chiefly a sensory nerve.

64. A 19-year-old man leaps from the third floor of his dormitory in an apparent suicide attempt. He is brought to the emergency department unconscious. He has visible head and lower extremity injuries. He has a pulse of 110 beats per minute but is apneic. What is the best airway management for this patient?

a. Nasotracheal intubation
b. Oral intubation
c. Oral intubation with head-chin lift
d. Tracheostomy
e. Intubation is not necessary for this patient.

65. A 21-year-old woman is stabbed in the chest by her boyfriend. She is brought to the emergency department for evaluation. Her blood pressure is 130/80 mmHg, and her pulse is 90 beats per minute. Physical examination reveals a single stab wound to the left fifth intercostal space in the midclavicular line. Neck examination is normal. Trachea is midline, and the jugular veins are not distended. She does have decreased breath sounds in the left lung fields. Which of the following diagnoses can be ruled out on the basis of the above information?
a. Large left hemothorax
b. Open pneumothorax
c. Pericardial tamponade
d. Rupture of the left main stem bronchus
e. Tension pneumothorax

66. A 41-year-old man suffers a traumatic amputation of three of his fingers in a meat slicer. He has no prior medical or surgical history. Which of the following modalities should be used to transport the amputated fingers with the patient?
a. Place in clean plastic bag and pack with dry ice.
b. Place in clean plastic bag filled with room temperature water.
c. Place in clean plastic bag in a chest filled with crushed ice and water.
d. Place in clean plastic bag filled with hot water.
e. Wrap the amputated fingers in sterile dry gauze.

67. A 19-year-old woman presents to the emergency department after sustaining an injury to her right eye while placing her contact lens. She has significant right eye pain. She has a prior medical history of seasonal allergies. Physical examination reveals a simple abrasion. Fluorescein testing is performed and reveals no evidence of a stained epithelial defect. This rules out the possibility of which of the following?
a. Bacterial infection
b. Iritis
c. Trauma
d. Viral infection
e. Ulcer

68. A 29-year-old man who works in a factory sustained a foreign body injury to his right eye when a piece of metal shot off a conveyer belt. He is brought to the emergency department for evaluation. Physical examination of the right eye reveals a metallic foreign body on the eye with an epithelial rust ring. What is the most useful instrument to remove this foreign body?
a. Cyanoacrylate glue
b. Eye burr
c. Eye spud
d. Fine needle tip
e. Sterile water and alcohol

69. A 37-year-old chemistry teacher sustains a chemical splash of acid to his right eye while attempting to perform a demonstration to his high school science class. He is in significant pain. While in the classroom and waiting for an ambulance to transport him to the hospital, which of the following interventions should be performed?
a. Eyedrop instillation with normal saline
b. Eye patch placement
c. Flush eye with 1 to 2 L of normal saline
d. Placement of eye under direct sunlight
e. Watchful waiting until ambulance arrives

70. A 37-year-old construction worker sustained a crush injury to his right thigh after a crane fell on his leg at the work site. He is brought to the emergency department for evaluation. He has significant right leg pain and pain with passive stretch. The leg is tense to palpation. What is the most likely intracompartmental pressure measurement of this patient's right leg?
a. 5 mm Hg
b. 10 mm Hg
c. 15 mm Hg
d. 25 mm Hg
e. 35 mm Hg

71. A 41-year-old woman who cleans houses for a living presents to her primary care physician complaining of tenderness in her right knee. The pain is constant and has been present for 3 weeks. She is in a monogamous relationship. Physical examination reveals that her knee is slightly swollen and tender. Cardiac, pulmonary, and abdominal examinations are within normal limits. A synovial aspiration is performed. The evaluation reveals no evidence of crystals or bacteria. What is the most likely diagnosis?
a. Bursitis
b. Infectious arthritis
c. Rheumatoid arthritis
d. Septic thrombophlebitis
e. Trauma-induced infectious arthritis

72. A 12-year-old boy who is the star pitcher of his little league team complains of right shoulder pain. This is his pitching arm. He has no prior medical or surgical history. Physical examination reveals weakness of the rotator cuff tendon. What is the most appropriate treatment for this patient?

a. Injection of corticosteroids
b. Intravenous corticosteroids
c. Rest, elevation, and anti-inflammatory agents
d. Sling placement
e. Surgical repair

73. A 65-year-old man with a history of coronary artery disease is undergoing an aortobifemoral bypass. Which of the following intraoperative management maneuvers will decrease his risk of intraoperative myocardial infarction?
a. Beta blockade
b. Calcium channel blockade
c. Administration of normal saline instead of lactated Ringer
d. Use of propofol
e. Use of morphine

74. A 35-year-old healthy man is diagnosed with an inguinal hernia. He has no history of abnormal bleeding. Which of the following tests is absolutely required prior to taking him to the operating room?
a. Hematocrit
b. Platelet count
c. Potassium
d. White blood cell count
e. None of the above

75. A 50-year-old man has diarrhea after an uncomplicated bowel resection. The fluid choice that most closely resembles his output is
a. Normal saline
b. Half normal saline with 20 mEq of potassium
c. D5W with 3 amp bicarbonate
d. Lactated Ringer
e. D5NS

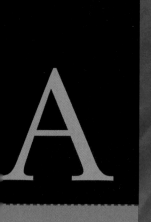

Answers

1. A (Chapter 2)

This patient likely has an abdominal aortic aneurysm. Ninety-five percent of aneurysms of the abdominal aorta are associated with atherosclerosis. This condition is responsible for approximately 15,000 deaths per year. Men are affected nearly 10 times more than women. Marfan syndrome can be associated with increased protease activity on histologic evaluation of the aneurysm wall. Syphilitic aneurysms occur in late-stage syphilis. Meningococcal infection is rarely associated with aneurysm formation. Trauma is a rare cause of abdominal aortic aneurysm.

2. E (Chapter 2)

This patient likely has acute mesenteric ischemia. Patients complain of sudden onset of abdominal pain with severe nausea, diarrhea, and/or vomiting. Pain is out of proportion to physical findings. Treatment involves surgical resection of infracted bowel as soon as possible. Aggressive surgical intervention should not be delayed because of the high index of suspicion of infracted bowel. Angiographic embolization may be diagnostic and therapeutic but is not considered a first-line therapy. Antibiotic therapy is considered an adjunctive therapy. Heparinization is not a first-line therapy for this condition.

3. C (Chapter 2)

A major portion of circulation for the lower extremity begins with the superficial femoral artery, which forms the popliteal artery passing behind the knee joint. This vessel then branches into the anterior tibial, posterior tibial, and peroneal arteries. There is no evidence to suggest rupture, hematoma, or spasm in these vessels. With knee injuries, the popliteal artery may go into spasm because of its location just posterior to the joint. It is important for practitioners to always palpate for a pulse in this artery in all patients with knee injuries. This vessel is also important, as it determines vascular supply to the distal leg.

4. D (Chapter 3)

Younger women have more fibrous tissue, which makes mammograms harder to interpret. Thus, ultrasound is a useful testing modality. As women age, breast tissue transforms from fibrous tissue to adipose tissue. This change makes it easier for mammography to detect masses. Thus, this modality is more useful in patients over the age of 35 years. Watchful waiting may be considered if the lesion is benign. Testing for the BRCA gene may be considered if the patient is suspect to a family history of breast cancer.

5. A (Chapter 3)

Women with mastitis need close follow-up for inflammatory breast disease. If a breast abscess developed, she would need antibiotics. If her breast abscesses were recurrent, the physician should consider resection of the involved ducts. If a patient with fibrocystic disease has straw-colored fluid on aspiration, she would need to be followed closely. If the patient had spontaneous galactorrhea, the physician would need to rule out a prolactinoma.

6. A (Chapter 3)

This patient should be treated with multiagent chemotherapy. This is the treatment of choice for a premenopausal patient with stage I or II breast cancer (size <1 cm), negative lymph nodes, and estrogen receptor status negative. Watchful waiting may be appropriate for patients with small tumors and negative lymph nodes. External beam radiotherapy is not indicated for this patient. High-energy focused ultrasound therapy is not indicated for the treatment of breast cancer. Tamoxifen is considered in patients who are estrogen receptor positive and have tumor size >1 cm.

7. B (Chapter 4)

This patient likely has ulcerative colitis. Colonoscopy may reveal thickened, friable mucosa. Fissures and pseudopolyps may also be present. This disease almost always involves the rectum and extends backward toward the cecum to varying degrees. Anoscopy is a limited procedure and will not allow visualization of the entire colon. Flexible or rigid sigmoidoscopy will allow visualization of the rectum and sigmoid colon but will miss higher levels of the colon. This patient requires further testing to establish a definitive diagnosis.

8. E (Chapter 4)

This patient has diverticulosis due to the presence of outpouchings in the wall of the colon that occur where the arterial supply penetrates the bowel wall. Patients who stop bleeding and are asymptomatic require no further treatment. Elective colectomy is not recommended at the first episode; thus, right hemicolectomy, left hemicolectomy, or subtotal colectomy are not required. Intravenous antibiotic therapy is not required in this patient, as there is no evidence of infection.

9. D (Chapter 4)

This patient has sigmoid volvulus. This condition can be reduced with a rectal tube, which is the treatment of choice. In addition, one can consider decompression with enema. Cecal calculus is treated with surgical intervention. High-fiber diet has no role in the treatment of volvulus. Lactulose is unlikely to be of benefit in the management of this patient.

10. E (Chapter 5)

This patient likely has a prolactinoma, the most common type of pituitary neoplasm. Women may present with headaches, irregular menses, amenorrhea, or galactorrhea. A serum prolactin level of >300 ug/L suggests the diagnosis of pituitary adenoma. This can be confirmed with MRI. Ferritin levels would likely be normal in this patient. Hemoglobin and hematocrit levels should be normal in this patient. Iron levels should be normal in this patient.

11. C (Chapter 5)

This patient would be expected to have fibroblast dysfunction. Patients with inflammatory bowel disease may require treatment with exogenous corticosteroids. These agents suppress the immune system and impair inflammatory cell migration. Antibody production is impaired. This is appropriate in Crohn disease. Other effects of corticosteroids include fibroblast dysfunction and impaired wound healing.

12. E (Chapter 5)

Renal failure is the most common cause of secondary hyperparathyroidism. This patient, who has had severe uncontrolled diabetes and lab values consistent in patients with diabetes, is most likely to have renal failure as the cause of his hypercalcemia. Whenever the kidney loses its ability to reabsorb calcium and hydroxylate vitamin D for calcium absorption from the gut, hypocalcemia triggers the parathyroid glands to increase their production of parathyroid hormone. Milk-alkali syndrome can cause hypercalcemia in patients who eat many antacids or drink an excessive amount of milk. This condition is more commonly found in patients who have gastric ulcers and frequently depend on milk and antacids for relief. Lithium can cause hypercalcemia by causing hyperparathyroidism. Parathyroid adenomas can cause hypercalcemia by increasing parathyroid hormone secretion.

13. A (Chapter 6)

The arcuate ligament does not inhibit gastroesophageal (GE) reflux and will not protect the esophageal mucosa from erosion. The esophagus limits its exposure to acid by several mechanisms, including salivation, gravity, gastric emptying, and the activity of peptic acid. Also important is the maintenance of a critical esophagogastric angle and appropriate diaphragmatic location of the GE junction.

14. B (Chapter 6)

This patient has diffuse esophageal spasm. Patients present with chest pain and dysphagia. Manometric studies reveal high-amplitude contractions and normal relaxation of the lower esophageal sphincter. Cricopharyngeal spasm occurs due to muscular dysfunction. Scleroderma is a collagen vascular disease that can affect the esophagus and cause motility dysfunction. Tuberculosis can be associated with esophageal diverticula of the traction type. This patient has no evidence to suggest a psychogenic swallowing disorder.

15. E (Chapter 6)

This child ingested a caustic alkaline substance. The child has difficulty breathing and has stridor. Airway edema is likely. Thus, tracheostomy should be performed first. Antibiotics and corticosteroids are secondary to the important primary survey of airway, circulation, and breathing in this patient. Vomiting should not be induced for a patient with a caustic ingestion. Likewise, placement of a nasogastric tube should be deferred.

16. A (Chapter 7)

This patient likely has cancer of the gallbladder. Eighty percent of cases are due to adenocarcinoma. Approximately 10% are anaplastic carcinoma, while 5% are squamous cell carcinoma. A right upper quadrant mass may be palpable. Signs of jaundice are also possible. This lesion is unlikely to be a sarcoma. Transitional cell carcinoma occurs in the urinary tract. Tuberculosis granuloma is found in the lung.

17. E (Chapter 7)

This patient has a type II cholesterol stone. This is produced as a result of homogeneous nucleation and can produce large gallstones. This type of gallstone represents 5% to 20% of all gallstones. Type 1 cholesterol stones are small in size and often multiple. Calcium oxalate stones are often found in the kidney. Black and brown gallstones are smaller in size and multiple in number.

18. A (Chapter 7)

This patient has the Charcot triad of fever, jaundice, and upper quadrant pain. This triad is seen with acute cholangitis. Initial treatment consists of fluid resuscitation and antibiotics. Patients who do not respond to this therapy need to be decompressed with percutaneous transhepatic drainage. T-tube decompression can also be considered if there is failure to respond to antibiotics. Choledochojejunostomy is considered when the bile duct is dilated.

19. B (Chapter 8)

This patient has evidence of aortic stenosis. Progressive degeneration and calcification of the valve leaflets occur. Patients can complain of angina, syncope, and dyspnea. A crescendo-decrescendo murmur can be heard best in the second right intercostal space. Electrocardiogram reveals left ventricular hypertrophy. Bundle branch block is uncommon, as is T wave inversion.

20. C (Chapter 8)

This patient has evidence of coronary artery disease that ultimately led to death. This is confirmed with the autopsy findings of myocardial necrosis and rupture of the left ventricle. Risk factors for coronary artery disease include hypertension, smoking, hypercholesterolemia, family history of heart disease, personal history of diabetes mellitus, and obesity. Atherosclerosis is the predominant pathogenic mechanism underlying obstructive disease of the coronary arteries.

21. C (Chapter 8)

This patient likely has a metastatic tumor to the heart. In this case, lymphoma is likely because of the following symptoms: fever, fatigue, weight loss, and an elevated white blood cell count beyond what would be expected with infection. Atrial myxoma would manifest as a mass lesion detectible with echocardiogram. Atrial fibrillation is unlikely given the findings presented. This patient has no colorectal symptoms; thus, metastatic colorectal carcinoma is unlikely. Pericarditis is unlikely given the presenting findings in this patient.

22. C (Chapter 9)

This newborn has omphalocele, an opening in the abdominal wall at the umbilicus that is due to incomplete closure of the somatic folds of the anterior abdominal wall in the fetus. The omphalocele can be a part of the pentalogy of Cantrell, which is associated with a diaphragmatic hernia, cleft sternum,

absent pericardium, intracardiac defects, and exstrophy of the bladder. Cleft lip and palate are not present in these patients.

23. E (Chapter 9)

The optimal time of convalescence after hernia repair is unknown. After traditional open surgery, patients have been asked to convalesce for 6 to 8 weeks. However, after laparoscopic mesh repair, patients may return to strenuous activity in 2 to 3 weeks. However, the true optimal time of convalescence is not known.

24. A (Chapter 9)

Femoral hernias are located in the femoral canal. The entrance to the canal is bounded superiorly and medially by the iliopubic tract, inferiorly by Cooper ligament, and laterally by the femoral vein. The inguinal ligament is more superficial. The ischial spine is not part of the femoral triangle. The lacunar ligament is not part of the femoral triangle. The femoral vein, not the femoral nerve, forms the lateral boundary of the triangle.

25. B (Chapter 10)

While preservation of the bladder neck, nervi erigentes, and the size of the bladder neck have all been associated with continence, the only factor that is generally accepted as being related to urinary control after radical prostatectomy is preservation of the external sphincter.

26. C (Chapter 10)

This patient presents with a residual bulky mass after three courses of platinum-based chemotherapy. While the chest x-ray and β hCG are normal, the serum AFP remains slightly elevated. AFP production is usually attributed to yolk sac elements in a mixed germ cell tumor. It is also seen with a number of other conditions, such as hepatocellular carcinomas and benign hepatic disease, including alcohol hepatitis, as is probable in this case. Patients with persistent marker elevations after chemotherapy are usually considered very likely to harbor residual carcinoma and probably best managed by further chemotherapy. However, the AFP elevation seen in this case is more likely due to benign liver disease. Consequently, this patient would be best managed by retroperitoneal lymph node dissection instead. The most likely finding at retroperitoneal lymph node dissection would be either fibrosis or residual teratoma. CT scan–directed percutaneous needle biopsy would have considerable sampling error, and external beam radiotherapy has no efficacy, particularly in the management of teratoma. Further observation is usually not warranted in patients who have residual retroperitoneal masses in excess of 2 to 3 cm.

27. A (Chapter 10)

The frequency of development of metachronous upper tract tumors in patients with superficial transitional cell carcinoma

(TCC) of the bladder is not exactly known but has been estimated to be very low (1%–3%). The incidence is higher in patients with higher stage (T2+) primary lesions (2%–8%). Patients treated for high-risk superficial TCC with BCG demonstrate a higher rate (13%–18%) of upper tract tumors over 3 years of follow-up. The best follow-up approach in patients treated with BCG is, therefore, the addition of upper tract imaging in the form of an intravenous pyelogram or CT urogram. Selective cytology as a routine practice is not recommended.

28. A (Chapter 11)

This patient likely has adenocarcinoma of the gallbladder, the most common pathology of gallbladder carcinoma. Ninety percent of patients have cholelithiasis. Metastases can occur to the lymph nodes and to the liver. Prognosis is poor and has a 5-year survival rate, ranging from 0% to 10%. There are several rare benign tumors of the gallbladder, including fibroma, lipoma, myxoma, and myoma.

29. A (Chapter 11)

This patient has a congenital malformation of the pancreaticobiliary tree. Specifically, this is a type U choledochal cyst, which is a fusiform dilation of the common bile duct. The type II cyst is a diverticulum of the common bile duct. The type III cyst is a choledochocele involving the bile duct within the liver. The type IV cyst is a cystic celation of the intrahepatic ducts. The type V cyst does not exist.

30. D (Chapter 11)

This patient has sustained a penetrating injury. Gallbladder injuries are uncommon but are seen after such trauma, as in this patient. When the gallbladder is injured, one must search for other injuries. The most frequent associated injury, in 72% of cases, is to the liver. Aortic injuries are less common than are liver injuries. Colon injuries are less common than are liver injuries. Kidney injuries are commonly associated with penetrating trauma. Urinary bladder trauma is often associated with pelvic fractures.

31. E (Chapter 12)

The combination of cough, hemoptysis, wheezing, and smoking history suggests the diagnosis of lung cancer. Of the two lung cancers listed, squamous cell carcinoma is the one that may produce parathyroid hormone (PTH)-related peptide protein. PTH receptor (PTHr) leads to hypercalcemia. Small cell carcinomas commonly produce antidiuretic hormone (ADH) or adrenocorticotropin hormone (ACTH). In a patient with Goodpasture, hemoptysis may present before hematuria, but because of the other symptoms, squamous cell carcinoma is the better choice. Renal cell carcinoma, not renal adenoma, may produce ectopic PTH-related protein (PTHrP), and smokers

do have an increased risk, but these patients present with hematuria, a palpable mass, flank pain, and a fever. The lack of an immunoglobulin G or A spike on serum protein electrophoresis should rule out multiple myeloma.

32. B (Chapter 12)

Laryngeal papillomas are benign neoplasms usually located on the true vocal cords. In children, they present as multiple lesions and are usually caused by human papilloma virus. In adults, they occur as single lesions and sometimes undergo malignant change. A singer's nodule is a small benign laryngeal polyp associated with chronic irritation from excessive use or heavy cigarette smoking and is usually found on the true vocal cords. Thyroid carcinoma is unlikely in children.

33. E (Chapter 12)

Squamous cell carcinoma is the most common type of cancer of the larynx. Cigarette smoking is the most important risk factor. Laryngeal polyps are small and benign. They are usually associated with chronic irritation from excessive use or heavy cigarette smoking. Mucoepidermoid and adenocarcinoma of the larynx are not as common as squamous cell carcinoma and don't have dysplasia as a precursor. Laryngitis is acute inflammation of the larynx, trachea, and epiglottis and is most often caused by a viral infection.

34. E (Chapter 13)

Phimosis is an acquired or congenital condition in which the foreskin cannot be pulled back behind the glans penis. In acquired phimosis, there likely is a history of poor hygiene, chronic balanoposthitis, or forceful retraction of a congenital phimosis. Balanitis is inflammation of the glans of the penis. Hypospadias is an anomaly in which the urethral meatus opens on the ventral surface of the penis. Epispadias is an anomaly in which the urethral meatus opens on the dorsal surface of the penis. Paraphimosis is an emergency condition in which the foreskin, once pulled back behind the glans penis, cannot be brought down to its original position.

35. C (Chapter 13)

Dutasteride is 5-alpha reductase inhibitor used in the symptomatic treatment of benign prostatic hyperplasia (BPH) that blocks the conversion of testosterone to dihydroxytestosterone (DHT) in target tissues. Because DHT is the major intracellular androgen in the prostate, dutasteride is effective in suppressing DHT and, subsequently, stimulation of prostatic growth and secretory function. Prostate size will decrease by approximately 25%. Ejaculatory dysfunction occurs in 5% to 8% of patients. Serum prostate-specific antigen (PSA) will decrease by 50%. AUA symptom scores typically improve by 5 to 7 points.

36. D (Chapter 13)

More than 90% of testicular tumors derive from germ cell tumors; the remainder are gonadal stromal tumors or metastatic from another site. The most common solid tumor in men between the ages of 15 and 40 is a seminoma. These tumors are typically confined to the testicle and associated with a hypoechoic area on ultrasound. This is an important feature, as most other testis tumors are associated with mixed echogenicity on ultrasound. Nonseminomatous germ cell tumors include embryonal carcinoma, choriocarcinoma, endodermal yolk sac tumor, and teratoma.

37. B (Chapter 14)

Arachnoid villi open at a pressure of 5 mm Hg. They act as one-way valves. Cerebrospinal fluid can be absorbed around the spinal nerve roots. Cerebrospinal fluid flows through the ventricles and exits by the foramen of Magendie. The total volume of cerebrospinal fluid is 150 mL.

38. C (Chapter 14)

Epidural hematoma results from hemorrhage into the potential space between the dura and the skull. The hemorrhage most likely results from rupture to a meningeal artery, which travels within this plane; the middle meningeal artery, which branches off the maxillary artery in the temporal area, is most common. Normally, the patient experiences a lucid interval, defined as an asymptomatic period of a few hours following the trauma. A Berry aneurysm results from a defect in the media of arteries and is usually located at bifurcation sites. Berry aneurysms are most commonly found in the circle of Willis. The source of bleeding due to subdural hematoma is from bridging veins; these often occur in the elderly due to minor trauma, and symptoms usually occur slowly—days to weeks. Bacterial meningitis diagnosis is confirmed with lumbar puncture and demonstrates increased neutrophils/protein and decreased glucose in the cerebrospinal fluid.

39. D (Chapter 14)

This patient may have an acoustic neuroma. These lesions arise from the vestibular portion of cranial nerve VIII. MRI has now become the method of choice for evaluation of posterior fossa and cerebellopontine angle tumors, because they are better seen on MRI as compared with CT. Audiometric testing is useful for lesions of cranial nerve VIII. Brainstem-evoked potential testing is useful for lesions of cranial nerve VIII. Nystagmography is useful for evaluation of vestibular disorders.

40. B (Chapter 15)

The most appropriate incision for a single lung transplant is via lateral thoracotomy. Double lung transplants are usually performed through a transverse anterior thoracotomy incision. Chevron incisions are useful for renal surgery. Midline abdominal incisions are appropriate for abdominal surgeries, not thoracic surgeries. Pfannenstiel incisions are appropriate to approach the female genitourinary tract.

41. C (Chapter 15)

One thing to consider after lung transplantation is survival. It is similar when comparing single to double lung transplantation. It is also related to diagnosis. The best survival is with obstructive lung disease. This is followed by cystic fibrosis. The worst survival is associated with pulmonary hypertension. Bronchogenic carcinoma also has a poor survival rate. Patients with lung cancer are not considered candidates for lung transplantation.

42. A (Chapter 15)

Most candidates for liver transplantation have end stage liver disease and are likely to die in 1 to 2 years. Children who require liver transplantation often have biliary atresia (in 50% of cases). In adults, postnecrotic cirrhosis accounts for 55% of cases, of which most are due to alcoholism or chronic hepatitis B. Approximately 15% of cases involve primary biliary cirrhosis and primary sclerosing cholangitis.

43. D (Chapter 16)

Pancreatic insufficiency, which is commonly seen in patients with cystic fibrosis, presents with malabsorptive issues and severe steatorrhea. Proper advice is to limit fat intake, as well as to increase ingestion of fat-soluble vitamins. Glucose malabsorption would not have such effects upon stooling. Menstrual loss could incur an anemic condition but not odorous stools. Bleeding ulcers can also cause anemia and black tarry stools, without the odor issues.

44. E (Chapter 16)

The exocrine pancreas is anastomosed to the bladder, and by measuring amylase, the exocrine product of the pancreas, one can monitor the functioning of the graft. Unless the patient had a pancreatectomy, the native pancreas may be making amylase. For the first several days postoperative, the serum glucose may not stabilize, and insulin may be required. The native pancreas may make a variably small amount of insulin, so direct measurement of the graft is not possible. The graft may have good blood flow but not be functioning well due to microvascular damage.

45. A (Chapter 16)

Ranson developed 11 criteria to determine the severity of pancreatitis. These factors are divided into admission criteria and initial 48-hours criteria. This patient's age of <55 years is reassuring. His blood glucose level is worrisome. His serum lactate dehydrogenase (LDH) level is worrisome. His serum calcium level is also worrisome. His serum calcium level is low and is also worrisome.

46. D (Chapter 17)

The superior parathyroid glands are located at the junction of the upper and middle third of the thyroid gland on the posteromedial aspect. The inferior parathyroids are located near the junction of the inferior thyroid and the recurrent laryngeal nerve. The carotid sinus is not near the location of the superior parathyroid glands.

47. E (Chapter 17)

Ultrasonography will define an enlarged parathyroid gland in 70% to 80% of cases. Dual tracer imaging can localize adenoma or hyperplasia in 70% of cases. Thyrocervical angiography is reserved for patients with recurrent hyperparathyroidism after surgical neck exploration. CT and MRI are helpful to locate enlarged parathyroid glands that are in the mediastinum.

48. C (Chapter 17)

This patient has tertiary hyperparathyroidism, which occurs in patients with chronic renal disease despite a successful renal transplant. Patients will have hypercalcuria (elevated urine calcium). There is no change in LDH levels. Serum phosphate levels are decreased. Serum and urine calcium levels are increased.

49. D (Chapter 18)

Melanocytes produce melanin and are chiefly responsible for pigmentation of the skin. They are of neural crest origin. One of the diseases associated with melanocytes is vitiligo, which is characterized by flat, well-demarcated zones of pigment loss. Keratinocytes produce keratin, which forms a waterproof layer. Langerhans cells are antigen-presenting cells. Merkel cells are epidermal cells that function in cutaneous sensation. Adipocytes are fat storage cells.

50. A (Chapter 18)

Basal cell carcinomas are the most common skin tumors. They tend to involve skin-exposed areas, most often in the head and neck. Grossly, they are characterized by a pearly papule with overlying telangiectatic vessels. The lower lip is actually the most common site for a tobacco user to develop squamous cell carcinoma. Malignant melanomas are the most likely primary skin tumors to metastasize systemically. Histiocytosis X (Langerhans cell histiocytosis) is caused by a proliferation of Langerhans cells, which are normally found in the epidermis. Seborrheic keratosis is a benign squamoproliferative neoplasm, associated with sunlight exposure. Fair-skinned persons are at increased risk. Depth of tumor correlates with risk of metastases.

51. D (Chapter 18)

A keloid is an abnormal proliferation of connective tissue with an abnormal arrangement of collagen. This abnormal proliferation looks very similar to a tumorlike scar. Keloids are much more common in African American individuals and usually follow some sort of trauma—in this case, the ear piercing. The spitz nevus can be confused with malignant melanoma. However, the lack of color change or change in size would make melanoma a little less likely. Also, this patient is much younger than the average age of patients who present with melanomatous lesions. Spitz nevus is also known as juvenile melanoma; because of its benign nature, this name is falling out of use. It is important to always think of melanoma when this type of lesion is seen and to order appropriate tests to rule it out. Molluscum contagiosum is a viral disease caused by the DNA poxvirus. It is contracted via direct contact, and its lesions are characteristically pink, umbilicated, and dome-shaped.

52. D (Chapter 19)

Ovarian cancer is an associated risk for women with Peutz-Jeghers syndrome. Granulosa cell tumor is the most common. This condition is not associated with cervical carcinoma. Hereditary renal cell carcinoma can be associated with Von Hippel-Lindau disease. Hamartomas are not associated with liver carcinoma or pancreatic carcinoma.

53. D (Chapter 19)

This patient has carcinoid syndrome, which is caused by the release of substances from a carcinoid tumor. The medical treatment for carcinoid syndrome is octreotide, a somatostatin analogue. Topical or intravenous corticosteroids are not beneficial for this patient. Furosemide is a loop diuretic used to treat fluid overload states. Tetracycline is an antibiotic and is not indicated in the treatment of carcinoid syndrome.

54. A (Chapter 19)

Appendicitis is predominantly seen in young adults. It causes right lower quadrant pain, nausea, vomiting, mild fever, and leukocytosis. The inflamed appendix may become gangrenous and perforate in 24 to 48 hours. Therefore, immediate appendectomy is standard treatment. Pancreatitis typically presents with epigastric pain radiating into the back, nausea, vomiting, and fever. Crohn disease and ulcerative colitis are inflammatory bowel diseases that typically present with long-standing diarrhea. They do not typically present in an acute fashion, as in this patient. Diverticulitis is predominantly found in the elderly and typically presents with left lower quadrant pain.

55. C (Chapter 20)

The left gastroepiploic artery runs through the gastrosplenic ligament to reach the greater omentum. The gastroduodenal artery and the right gastric artery branch off of the common hepatic artery. The gastroduodenal artery descends behind the first part of the duodenum. The right gastric artery runs to the pylorus and then along the lesser curvature of the stomach. The left gastric artery and the splenic artery arise from the celiac trunk. The left gastric artery runs upward and to the left toward the cardia, giving rise to esophageal and hepatic branches, and then turns right and runs along the lesser curvature within the lesser omentum to anastomose with the right gastric artery.

56. C (Chapter 20)

This child has a Meckel diverticulum, which is a congenital anomaly resulting from an unobliterated yolk stalk. More specifically, it is a vestigial remnant of the omphalomesenteric duct. It presents as an ileal outpouching typically located close to the ileocecal valve. The presence of inflammation, ulceration, and gastrointestinal bleeding due to the presence of ectopic acid–secreting gastric epithelium is seen in approximately half of these patients. Remember the rule of 2s with Meckel diverticulum: It occurs in about 2% of children, occurs within approximately 2 ft of the ileocecal valve, contains 2 types of ectopic mucosa (gastric and pancreatic), and its symptoms usually occur by age 2.

57. C (Chapter 20)

Due to the symptoms of decreased burning with food intake and weight gain, a preliminary differential diagnosis of *Helicobacter pylori* would be appropriate. Treatment with the triple therapy of bismuth salicylate, metronidazole, and an antibiotic such as amoxicillin would be in order. The presentation of *Escherichia coli* tends to be a more acute infection. *E. coli* is associated with bloody diarrhea, and *Shigella* with abdominal cramping and diarrhea.

58. E (Chapter 21)

Thrombocytopenia is not a complication of a splenectomy. Thrombocytosis is a possible complication postsplenectomy. Anemia is not a direct result of splenectomy. Patients are unlikely to have basophilia or eosinophilia. Subphrenic abscess, atelectasis, pancreatitis, gastric dilation, and sepsis are the possible complications of splenectomy.

59. C (Chapter 21)

The peripheral blood smear in a postsplenectomy patient will show Pappenheimer bodies, Howell-Jolly bodies, and Heinz bodies. Nucleated red blood cells are found in the blood of sickle cell patients. Basophilic stippling is found in the blood of patients with lead poisoning. Spherocytes are found in patients with hemolytic anemia. Blister cells are found in the blood of patients with glucose-6-phosphate deficiency.

60. D (Chapter 21)

Postsplenectomy patients should receive vaccinations against encapsulated organisms. The common encapsulated organisms are *Streptococcus pneumoniae*, *Neisseria meningitides*, and *Haemophilus influenzae*. The best time to vaccinate these patients is preoperatively.

61. B (Chapter 22)

This patient likely has Hashimoto thyroiditis. Patients have mild thyroid tenderness and fatigue. Laboratory features include the presence of thyroid autoantibodies. Frequently, no treatment is necessary for this condition. Acute thyroiditis is associated with fever, chills, and dysphagia. Papillary carcinoma is associated with a palpable thyroid nodule. Riedel thyroiditis is associated with thyroid fibrosis. Symptoms of tracheal and esophageal compression are possible.

62. E (Chapter 22)

This patient has evidence of papillary carcinoma of the thyroid. Only 5% of patients with papillary carcinoma of the thyroid present with distant metastases. For tumors that are <1.5 cm and that are disease-confined to one lobe and no extracapsular extension, treatment with thyroid lobectomy is appropriate. External beam radiotherapy is not required for this patient. Multiagent chemotherapy is not required for this patient. Subtotal and total thyroidectomy are not required for this patient.

63. A (Chapter 22)

Injury to the nerve causes bowing of the vocal cords during phonation. This can be a problem in singers who have difficulty reaching high-pitched notes. The nerve can be at risk during thyroid surgical procedures because of its proximity to the superior thyroid artery. The nerve is both sensory and motor to the larynx.

64. D (Chapter 23)

This patient is apneic. An airway must be established for this patient. However, he may also have fractures of the cervical spine. Thus, the best treatment for this patient in terms of airway management is a tracheostomy. Nasotracheal intubation is inappropriate for a patient who is totally apneic. Oral intubation and oral intubation with head-chin lift is inappropriate because it requires some hyperextension of the neck. Intubation is necessary for a patient who is apneic.

65. B (Chapter 23)

It is unlikely that this patient has an open pneumothorax. Patients with pneumothorax are in obvious respiratory distress. They often have an obvious "sucking" chest wound. This patient has neither of the above findings. Left pneumothorax is possible in this patient and needs evaluation with a chest x-ray. Cardiac tamponade is possible in this patient, as is rupture of the main stem bronchus. Tension pneumothorax is also a consideration for this patient.

66. C (Chapter 23)

An amputated upper extremity body part can be replanted if properly recovered and transported with the patient. Cooling the body part in a chest filled with crushed ice and water may preserve the body part for up to 18 hours. The body part should not be placed in dry gauze or packed with dry ice. In addition, the body part should not be placed in warm water.

67. E (Chapter 23)

An ulcer will appear as a fluorescein-stained epithelial defect with a local corneal infiltrate. This patient appears to have no evidence of an ulcer. However, this form of testing does not rule out the presence of bacterial infection, iritis, trauma, or viral infection. This patient will benefit from treatment with quinolone eyedrops and avoidance of eye patching. Close follow-up with a physician is also recommended.

68. B (Chapter 23)

This patient has suffered a metallic foreign body to the eye with an epithelial rust ring. These should be removed immediately with an eye burr. Foreign bodies of the cornea can also be approached with a fine needle tip or an eye spud. Sterile water may be utilized, but alcohol exposure to the eye should be avoided. Cyanoacrylate glue adheres to the eyes and should also be avoided.

69. C (Chapter 23)

This patient has sustained a chemical burn to the eye. The eye should be immediately flushed at the scene with 1 to 2 L of normal saline, which should be continued in the emergency department. A topical anesthetic and a Morgan lens will facilitate flushing. Eye patch placement is not indicated. Placement of the eye under direct sunlight may damage the eye. Watchful waiting is not recommended; this patient needs eye lavage as soon as possible.

70. E (Chapter 25)

This patient likely has a compartment syndrome, which is caused by an increase in interstitial fluid pressure within an osteofascial compartment, leading to compromise of the microcirculation and myoneural necrosis. Diagnosis is confirmed by an intracompartmental pressure of 30 mm Hg or higher. Treatment of this condition is surgical fascial release.

71. A (Chapter 25)

Bursae are fluid-filled sacs that cushion areas of friction between tendon and bone or skin. Bursae are lined with special cells called synovial cells, which secrete a fluid rich in collagen and proteins. This synovial fluid acts as a lubricant when parts of the body move. When this fluid becomes irritated because of too much movement, the painful condition known as bursitis results. Rheumatoid arthritis is a multisystem disorder that results in symmetrical joint inflammation, articular erosions, and extra-articular complications. Infectious arthritis is unlikely in the absence of joint fluid aspiration that reveals an organism. Septic thrombophlebitis is unlikely given the history of this patient. Trauma is also unlikely given the history of this patient.

72. C (Chapter 25)

This patient may have suffered a tear of the rotator cuff. Most tears are small and may be treated symptomatically with rest, elevation, and anti-inflammatory agents. If the shoulder still demonstrates pain after a trial of conservative therapy, surgical repair should be considered. Injection of corticosteroids or intravenous corticosteroids is not considered to be first-line therapy for this patient.

73. A (Chapter 26)

Multiple randomized controlled studies have demonstrated decreased mortality and morbidity with intraoperative beta blockade in high-risk patients. This is one of the few interventions that has been clearly shown to improve outcomes.

74. E (Chapter 26)

In the setting of a normal history and physical, it is not necessary to obtain preoperative labs for minor surgery, though many surgeons and institutions will do this.

75. D (Chapter 26)

Lactated Ringer is a bicarbonate-rich solution with an electrolyte composition similar to stool output.

Index

Page numbers followed by *f* refer to illustrations; page numbers followed by *t* refer to tables.

Hematoma
   epidural, 99, 99*f*
   subdural, 100, 100*f*
Hematuria
   in bladder cancer, 68
   in kidney cancer, 68
Hemolytic anemias, 155
Hemoptysis
   in lung cancer, 80
   in mitral stenosis, 58
Hemorrhage
   gastrointestinal, 32
   in immune thrombocytopenic
      purpura, 154–155
   in portal hypertension, 74–75
   spleen, 153–154
   in stress ulceration, 146
   subarachnoid, 97–99, 98*f*
   in trauma patient, 167
Hemothorax, 167
Hepatocellular adenoma, 71
Hepatocellular carcinoma, 72, 72*f*
Hepatoma, 72
Hernia
   epidemiology, 62
   femoral, 63, 192, 201
   inguinal, 62–63, 63*f*, 187
   locations, 63, 64*f*
   obturator, 63
   postoperative recovery time, 192, 201
   umbilical, 63
HIDA scan, 52
Hip fracture, 180
Histamine-2 blockers
   for gastric and duodenal ulcers, 145
   for gastrinoma, 147
Hoarseness, 162, 193, 202
Hodgkin disease, staging, 155
Horizontal mattress suture, 7*f*
Hormones
   adrenal, 39–40, 50*f*
   pituitary, 37, 38*f*
Horner syndrome, 80
Howell-Jolly bodies, 196, 205
Howship-Romberg sign, 63
Human leukocyte antigen (HLA), 106
Hyaluronic acid injection, 178
Hyperacute rejection, 106
Hyperaldosteronism, 41
Hypercalcemia, 121–124, 123*t*, 190, 200
Hyperkalemia, 185
Hypernatremia, 185
Hyperparathyroidism, 121–124, 123*t*, 194, 204
Hypersplenism, 155
Hypertension
   in hyperaldosteronism, 41
   in pheochromocytoma, 42
   portal, 45
Hyperthyroidism, 159–161

Hypocalcemia, 121, 124
Hypokalemia
   in hyperaldosteronism, 41
   postoperative, 185
Hyponatremia, 185
Hypospadias, 202
Hypotension
   in aortic dissection, 14
   in thoracic aortic aneurysm, 13
   in trauma patient, 167

I
Ileocecal resection, 138, 138*f*
Immune thrombocytopenic purpura, 154–155
Immunosuppression, 106
Incisional hernia, 63, 64*f*
Infections, surgical site. *See* Surgical site infections
Inferior mesenteric artery, 26, 27*f*
Infliximab, 27
Inguinal hernia, 62–63, 63*f*
Insulin
   pancreatic secretion, 111–112
   perioperative management, 184
Interleukin-2, 68
Intracranial aneurysm, 97–99, 98*f*
Intraductal papilloma, 21
Intraoperative management
   anesthetics, 3
   antibiotics, 183, 183*t*
   blood products, 183
   cardiac risk factors, 183
   diabetes management, 183
   fluids and electrolytes, 183
   operating room environment, 3
   skin tension lines, 2*f*, 3
   temperature, 183
Intravenous pyelography
   in benign prostatic hyperplasia, 87
   in kidney cancer, 68
   in kidney stone disease, 67
Iodide, in Graves disease, 161
Irinotecan, 80
Iris scissors, 4, 4*f*
Ischemia, mesenteric, 16–17
Islets of Langerhans, 11

J
Jaundice, in portal hypertension, 74
Joint pain, 178–179

K
Keloid, 195, 204
Kidneys
   anatomy, 66
   cancer, 68
   stone disease, 66–67, 67*f*, 123
   transplantation, 108–109, 108*t*, 109*t*

Klebsiella
   in cholecystitis, 51
   in empyema, 84
   in liver abscess, 73
Knee injury, 189, 199
Knee pain, 179
Knife blades, 3–4, 4*f*
Kupffer cells, 70

L
Lactated Ringer, 185*t*, 206
Lactic dehydrogenase, 92
Laminectomy, 103, 104
Laryngeal nerve, 158, 159*f*
Larynx, cancer, 193, 202
Left ventricular hypertrophy, 57
Lentigo maligna melanoma, 129, 129*f*
Lesch-Nyhan syndrome, 66
Lidocaine, 3, 3*t*
Liver
   abscess, 73, 73*f*
   anatomy and physiology, 70, 71*f*
   benign tumors, 71
   cancer, 72, 72*f*
   transplantation, 107–108, 107*t*, 194, 203
Local anesthetics, 3, 3*t*
Lumbar disc disease, 103–104, 104*f*
Lumpectomy, 23
Lung
   anatomy, 77, 78*f*, 79*f*
   benign tumors, 77
   cancer, 78–82, 81–82*t*, 193, 202
   empyema, 84
   mesothelioma, 82
   pneumothorax, 83, 83*f*
   transplantation, 194, 203
   tumors with malignant potential, 77–78
Luteinizing hormone, hypersecretion, 39
Luteinizing hormone-releasing hormone (LH-RH) agonists, 91
Lymphadenopathy, 22
Lymphoma, 191, 201

M
Macroadenoma, pituitary, 37–38
Magnetic resonance angiography, 15
Magnetic resonance cholangiopancreatography, 53
Magnetic resonance imaging (MRI)
   in aortic aneurysm, 12
   in aortic dissection, 14
   in brain tumors, 97
   in colorectal cancer, 31
   in hyperaldosteronism, 41
   in liver cancer, 72
   in meningioma, 97
   in pheochromocytoma, 42